# WHAT KIND OF LIFE

# WHAT KIND OF LIFE

## THE LIMITS OF MEDICAL PROGRESS

DANIEL CALLAHAN

Georgetown University Press, Washington, D.C.

Georgetown University Press, Washington, D.C. 20007
© 1990 by Georgetown University Press. All rights reserved.
Originally published by Simon & Schuster, 1990.
Printed in the United States of America.
10  9  8  7  6  5  4  3  2                    1994
THIS VOLUME IS PRINTED ON ACID-FREE OFFSET BOOK PAPER.


**Library of Congress Cataloging-in-Publication Data**

Callahan, Daniel, 1930–
    What kind of life : the limits of medical progress / Daniel
Callahan.
        p.   cm.
    Includes bibliographical references and index.
    1. Medical care—United States. 2. Medical economics—United
States. 3. Medicine—Research—United States. 4. Medical ethics—
United States.    I. Title.
RA395.A3C324   1995
362.1′01—dc20
ISBN 0-87840-573-9 (pbk.)                           94-34440

For Sidney
and for
John C. Bennett
Agnes Bourneuf
John T. Edsall
Otto Guttentag
Marion Cahill Heffernan

# CONTENTS

# PREFACE

As a child in the 1930s, I spent a good deal of my time in the offices of doctors and the operating rooms of hospitals. For reasons I never learned, I was subject to recurrent infections, which went from my arms or legs to my lymph nodes. The only cure in those days was to lance the nodes and allow them to drain. Time and again I was dragged, screaming and struggling, to an operating room where an ether mask was forced over my face; the sense of smothering was palpable. I awoke, vomiting, to face weeks of bed rest and the painful daily changing of bandages.

I mention this not to indulge in the bittersweet pleasure of exchanging illness stories, but to mark how much our medical lives have changed since then, and to make clear my own subsequent debt to that medical progress I will so persistently question in this book. My children underwent no such ordeals when they were growing up. Antibiotics took care of their infections. My own later, adult experiences with surgery no longer required that I be held down to have ether administered. The only good thing to be said of earlier times, which few are inclined to think of as the good old days, is that the cost of my treatments was minimal. My parents worried about me, but they did not have to worry about the expenses of my care.

Since then, everything has improved in the scientific practice of medicine, and I can testify personally to some of those benefits. What has not improved are the costs of that care. They remain out of control, steadily rising at an annual rate approximately twice that of general inflation. The $550 billion that we spend in this country on healthcare is not just a large number. It reflects the pressure of high costs that we are all now feeling—whether as elderly individuals, who have to pay more out of their pocket than in 1965, when Medicare was passed, or as employers, faced with insurance increases of anywhere from 20 to 70 percent over the past couple of years, or as young people, worried about the possibility of a catastrophic illness with its no less catastrophic costs. My children will, as a result, think twice before they even have children and, once they do, may well, despite some insurance, pay comparatively more out of pocket than my parents did nearly six decades ago.

What has happened here and why? What should we make of that situation? This book is an attempt to answer those questions. As I write it, there is fresh talk of national health insurance, and a number of groups have come forward with proposals for some system of minimally adequate care for all. These proposals come on top of others for improved long-term and home-care programs for the elderly, and improvements in the health of children; and of course, they come in the ongoing context of long-standing pleas for more research money, enough to help us cure those diseases that now cost so much.

Yet as valid as many of those proposals are, I have come to be profoundly uneasy about the adequacy of those plans to deal with the full problem of healthcare, particularly in the future. I am concerned less about the immediate economic viability of the new schemes than I am about their deeper premises, less about the possible techniques of financing decent healthcare than about the way we think about health in our lives. Why have past reform schemes failed? The usual answer is because we lack the political will or economic skills to make them work. I have become restless with that answer; it no longer seems adequate. I believe, instead, that the problem lies in our success rather than in our failure, our goals rather than our means, our ideals rather than our defects.

We have come to ever more desire what we cannot any longer have in unlimited measure—a healthier, extended life—and cannot even afford to pursue much longer without harm to our personal lives and our other social institutions. If we are to have any hope of finding a long-lasting solution to our health-care crisis, we must start by taking a hard look at that desire, one I share along with everyone else. For perhaps the healthcare problem is not quite what appears on the surface, just a matter of improved financing, equity, and efficiency. Perhaps it is a crisis about the meaning and nature of health, and about the place that the pursuit of health should have in our lives. Any serious consideration of healthcare must, in any case, begin with that basic issue, one we thought was long ago answered and solved.

One reason I have been led to begin there is because I do not share the inveterate optimism that seems a kind of virus in much discussion of healthcare, and certainly in its politics. It is the kind of virus that produces confident assertions that, if Canada can do it, so can we; or that, if we can just cut waste, we can afford whatever we need; or that we are beginning to turn the corner on cost containment; or that more research money will cure those expensive diseases that are such a drain on the system; or that it doesn't matter how much we spend on health anyway, because health is such a good thing and healthcare such a good employer. I look instead at the projections of future healthcare costs, all of which are enormous, and take them seriously. I see no reason to believe in magic fixes, whether scientific, bureaucratic, or financial. The projections tell me that we are going to have to change, and change not just the mechanics of our system, but our way of thinking about and understanding illness, life, health, and death. I see no reason why we cannot have a perfectly adequate system if we are prepared to do that. It will just have to be very different.

In 1987, I published *Setting Limits: Medical Goals in an Aging Society*, a book somewhat notorious for its dour assessment of our future ability to make the elderly more and more happy by spending more and more on their healthcare, and no less dour in judging that we could not economically afford to do so anyway. I was asked by some, "Why did you pick on the elderly?" The answer is that, in attempting to provide ever-improved healthcare for the elderly, we are on the greatest, and most extensive, of medicine's many frontiers of progress. It was as much a study of how to respond to such a frontier as it was a book about the elderly. This book is an attempt to look at the other frontiers, for it is quite true that it is our whole system that is in turmoil, not just our attempt to provide for those who are aged. For some readers of my earlier writings, there will be a few familiar themes—my concern with technology, individualism, and the setting of limits, for instance—themes that go back to my 1973 book, *The Tyranny of Survival*. It was then I first took up in a systematic way the moral and social problems of our national dedication to medical progress. *Setting Limits* was another stage along the way.

The subject of this book is the most daunting, and the task overwhelming in its power to intimidate. My aim is to set forth an alternative way of thinking about health that will lead into the devising of a reasonable and just healthcare system. I want it to be deeply rooted in a plausible understanding of the human condition and to be coherent, feasible, and humane in its practical policy implications. I have come, however, to think that no system can be perfectly reasonable, decent, and just. Any system in the future will always be an approximation, better or worse, but never perfect. I am acutely aware also that we begin *in medias res,* in the middle of the story, with a hardy, deeply ingrained set of values, a complex set of institutions, and a bewildering array of mores, folkways, interests, and predilections already in place. They will not be easy to change.

I am, however, trying once again to think forward over a period of the next ten to thirty years, and a great change in our values and institutions is possible over a period that long. The cultural shifts wrought by the civil rights movement, by feminism and environmentalism, by the neoconservative upsurge, and by the sexual revolution are not, historically, much farther back in our own history than that. They show us how malleable we are as a people, especially when we have become convinced change is necessary. I am not, then, disturbed by suggesting changes that will take many years to fully accomplish, and I am not deterred by likely criticisms that what I propose is not, at the moment, practical. In a recent Louis Harris poll, a remarkably high 89 percent of Americans polled said that they think the American healthcare system needs fundamental change.[1] That suggests to me the time is perfect to begin the long and difficult task of bringing about that change.

My question is this: How can we now begin making changes that will serve us well *in the long run,* even if they require some years to take root? I am concerned also that we will, in our desperation to deal with present problems, put into place solutions that will fall apart within a few years because of their failure to take account of the deeper causes of our problems. If we are not able to fully understand our present and future demands, we are likely to devise, once more, patchwork solutions that will delude us from looking at the harder problems and send us in directions that we will come to regret.

There are many ways to write books, and I have tried here to look at the problem of healthcare in a whole and entire kind of way, from beginning to end, so to speak. I have aimed to carry the problem through from philosophical premises to general policy recommendations, in great part because efforts of that kind seem in short supply. But the only way that goal seemed feasible was to think of the book as a kind of elaborate outline, an extended sketch, rather than a detailed blueprint; in another era, I might have called it a prolegomenon. Put another way, I have tried to paint a mural rather than a microscopically detailed miniature. I am seeking coherence and wholeness, even at the cost of failing to explore in needed detail the many difficulties and puzzles the discerning reader will readily discover. Our American penchant for muddling through, for distrusting long-term goals and visions, particularly fails us in confronting the dilemmas of healthcare. Piecemeal approaches accumulate knots and tangles, which then prove all but impossible to pull apart. Our first requirement is, therefore, to see if we can find a new purchase on old troubles, and that is what I have attempted.

Now it would be pretentious to think that I have come up with something wholly new, some *ex nihilo* creation. More than once, on the contrary, I have thought of myself as a type of aspiring chef, but one who keeps discovering that all new recipes seem to have more or less the same range of ingredients as the old ones, even though now and then someone will think of something new to add. In this case, many of the ingredients have been around for a long time, even though some have been neglected of late (an emphasis on public health, for instance), and I have tried to add a few new ones, hoping that the result will add something fresh to the debate. All of this is to say that I am indebted to the large number of people who have written on these topics over the years, or spoken at the many conferences and meetings I have attended. I am also anxious that I may not have given credit where appropriate. Every author on any important and much-debated topic will have at least one reader who will say, correctly enough, "But I said that ten years ago." I apologize in advance to that reader if I have failed to acknowledge my indebtedness.

Most generally, I have profited greatly from the imaginative and thoughtful writings of Rudolph Klein, professor of social policy at the University of Bath, a debt that is detailed in my notes. His writings on the British National Health Service are a model of social and policy analysis. My participation in an important project on health promotion sponsored by the Henry J. Kaiser Family Foundation has been illuminating. More specifically, and identifiably, I am indebted to a number of people who have read portions of this manuscript. They include, first and foremost, my colleague Courtney Campbell, editor of the *Hastings Center Report*, who used his own time to read each and every draft of each and every chapter. His help was astute and invaluable. Paul Menzel gave me the great advantage of his many years of thinking about ethics and medical economics and the chance to read the manuscript of his important new book, *Strong Medicine: The Ethical Rationing of Health Care* (Oxford University Press). Ruth Hanft, a shrewd and well-seasoned observer of American healthcare, gave advice at some critical junctures. Alexander Leaf, Marshall B. Kapp, Leslie Rothenberg, David Hadorn, and Thomas Wickizer all read various portions and their comments were insightful. My colleagues Bruce Jennings, Kathleen Nolan, and Susan Wolf also read sections of the book and were exceedingly helpful. Willard Gaylin, with whom I have talked about these issues over many years, was as usual a great source of insight and support, and Paul Homer, assistant director of The Hastings Center, helped to make my administrative chores more tolerable. Marna Howarth, Varun Gauri, and Sarah Swenson provided invaluable library help. Ellen McAvoy provided her usual loyal and diligent support, as did other colleagues at the Center.

I have dedicated this book to six people. Five of them have in common both advanced age and great wisdom, and my own life has been much enriched by my conversations and correspondence with them on the themes of this book and those of *Setting Limits*. They are what I aspire to be, and they have carried into their later years all the vigor of mind and spirit that gave them such distinguished careers. John C. Bennett is president emeritus of Union Theological Seminary, Agnes Bourneuf for many years managed a wonderful bookstore in Harvard Square, John T. Edsall is professor emeritus of biology at Harvard, Otto Guttentag, M.D., is professor emeritus of medicine at the University of California, San Francisco Medical School, and Marion Cahill Heffernan is a retired economist and educator.

The book is also dedicated to my wife, Sidney, a wonderful and thoughtful person. She was a constant help as I tried to think through the issues of this book. There must be nicer topics for husbands and wives to discuss during their evening walks than disease and sickness, but Sidney has never complained. Perhaps, though, that was better than the earlier walks, which had concentrated on aging and death. Some couples have all the fun.

# CHAPTER 1

# FROM EXPLOSION TO IMPLOSION: TRANSFORMING HEALTHCARE

Early in December of 1987, Adam Jacoby "Coby" Howard of Rockwood, Oregon, died of leukemia. His death came in the midst of a campaign by his family, friends, and teachers to raise $100,000 for a bone-marrow transplant. The campaign still had $30,000 to go at the time of his death. A year earlier there would have been no need for such an effort. The state of Oregon would have paid for the transplant. But Coby had the misfortune of being the first victim of a new, 1987 policy set by the Oregon legislature: to stop all organ transplantation for welfare recipients and spend the money instead on prenatal care. His aunt, Susan McGee, said, "We spent precious time fiddling around trying to raise money for the operation while Coby was dying . . . Coby himself spent some of his last days going around helping collect the donation cans."[1]

What was remarkable about this event was not that a child died because he had failed to get government support for a transplant. That had happened before, but usually before the states had mandated coverage for organ transplants, when they were still classified as experimental forms of therapy. Nor was it remarkable that there had been a rationing of medical resources.

17

Millions of Americans have long been denied critical care if they lacked money to pay for it. What was new was the openness of the decision, and the clear visibility of its victims. Instead of the kind of soft, covert rationing that has long been part of the American scene—either by the impersonal forces of the market or by the quiet, hidden way of parsimonious bureaucrats—there was a hard and open setting of priorities. Those denied treatment had faces.

The money needed for transplants, it was decided and publicly announced, would go to expectant mothers. That priority would be, so the argument went, a better investment of scarce funds. Many more of them could be helped, some 1,500 in all, compared with a handful of likely organ recipients. It was not, on the face of it, a casual or thoughtless decision. On the contrary, since the voters of Oregon had decidedly insisted that there be a strict and tough limit on state expenditures, there was no choice but for some difficult decisions to be made. A new and disturbing chapter had been opened in American healthcare. As Dr. John Kitzhaber, president of the Oregon Senate (and a physician, as it happens), noted, "Medical technology has outstripped, and will continue to outstrip, our ability to pay for it. . . . The cold reality is that . . . we must limit the money we spend on health care."[2]

Was Dr. Kitzhaber right? Many would say no. They could point out that there was a $200 million surplus in the Oregon state budget at the time. The transplant crisis was provoked by a voter-inspired expenditure limit that need not have happened and could be reversed in the future. They could in addition point out that millions of dollars are wasted, in Oregon and elsewhere, on cosmetics, expensive automobiles, VCRs, high-priced restaurants, and wasteful government programs. They could, moreover, note that just to the north, in the state of Washington, transplants remained available to welfare recipients. Even farther north, in Canada, they were available as well, and in a country that provides decent healthcare coverage for all of its citizens, regardless of their ability to pay. Its citizens can have both prenatal treatment and organ transplants. As if to rub it in, the Canadians make such treatment available while spending only 8.5 percent of their GDP (equivalent to our GNP) in 1986 on healthcare, compared with the 11.1 percent spent in the United States during that same year—and up to 11.5 percent now. That seems to underscore all the more the seemingly needless tragedy of the Oregon situation. Coby might not have had to die.

I suspect that is true, but to come to that conclusion is to choose the smaller, more poignant truth over the larger, more penetrating one. The larger truth lies with Dr. Kitzhaber's observation: We will not indefinitely continue to have the ability to pay for an expanding healthcare system, or for those endlessly emerging marvels of technology that promise to extend life. Some places will feel the pinch before others, and some will find temporary solutions better than others. Yet even if we can continue for a time to find the money to pay for organ transplants, or other yet-to-be-devised technologies, there is every reason to think that time is running out on the expansive, and expensive, enterprise of contemporary medicine. To talk about our "ability to pay" is itself misleading. If we are prepared to sacrifice other things necessary for a good society, if we want to spend most of what we have on health, then we can no doubt continue expanding indefinitely.

Yet if we begin to ask about the wisdom of that kind of unending medical progress, about the proper place of health among our whole range of social needs, and about the most responsible way to invest our money in the future, we may, and should, hesitate. In too many of our cities the hospital is the newest, best-equipped building, while the public school is the oldest, worst-equipped. Is that a good way to the future? Is that the right way to distribute our resources? We know and pity the hypochondriac, ever fearful of illness and death, ever willing to become absorbed to the point of obsession in a concern for health. We have yet to learn how to note the same characteristics in a society, one that has perhaps come to give a damaging priority to health needs, both real and imaginary. What should we think of the reported trend of Americans to feel sicker when their health is actually improving? What are we to make of the fact that contemporary Americans, the healthiest people in the history of the human race, are reported to believe that good health is the most important goal in their lives?[3] Ought that to be the most important goal for a life?

As we begin asking these larger questions, we will soon find ourselves moving uncomfortably in two realms. There is the intimate realm of individual people with names and faces, one of whom was called "Coby," and there is the larger, more impersonal and statistical realm of all of us together. As individuals we have come to need expensive organ transplants to make it through childhood, or costly bypass surgery to give us a few more years as elderly people. In our common life together as a society, however, we need those things that make for a public good: schools, highways, housing, parks, good police and fire protection. We are only now beginning to see that we cannot have it all. We cannot pursue medical advances wherever they lead us. We cannot give each individual what he or she may want or need to live some version of optimal health and longevity and, at the same time, have everything else needed to make a good society.

## LOOKING FOR A WAY OUT

Our first impulse is likely to be a rejection of what will seem a stark and tragic choice. We will say that we have simply failed to manage our more than ample resources well enough, or that we are as taxpayers too selfish, or that we do not value the life of individual persons as much as we should. We will invoke the glories of greater efficiency as a way out, and whenever there is a claim that too much is being spent on healthcare, we will seek (and probably find) some other sector which appears just as profligate. We can, then, find ways to continue business as usual. If we are liberals, we can lay the blame at the feet of those unwilling to support an equitable national healthcare system. If we are of a more conservative bent, we can always claim that government regulation has hindered the market from delivering the quality and equality of which it is so splendidly capable.

My goal in this book is to show that we have a more difficult problem on our hands, that the standard nostrums of neither right nor left will any longer suffice to cope with the problem before us. That problem can be directly stated: The very nature of medical progress is to pull to itself many more resources than should rationally be spent on it, often more than can be of genuine benefit to many individuals, and much, much more than can be socially justifiable for the common good.

The power of medical progress feeds off of a potent dynamic, by now well recognized. There is the increasing weight of an aging society, one that sees the elderly as the fastest-growing age group, and with that growth a sharp upward curve through intensified treatment in meeting healthcare pressures. There is the force of technological advancement, ever ingenious in finding new ways to improve and extend life, many of them as attractive as they are expensive. There is, most of all, the power of public demand, which has come to expect medicine to improve not only health but life more generally, and which has come to see a longer and better life as not simply a benefit but as a deep and basic right.

The combined force of that dynamic has resulted in an explosion of healthcare costs; it is a force that shows no sign of abating in this country and it will probably come to threaten the healthcare systems of other, better managed countries as well. That force is intensified by some important collateral forces. Among them are the great profitability of the American healthcare system for many thousands of people, where doing good and doing well have become synonymous; the individualism of our culture, which stimulates a steady escalation of need and desire; and the drive for equality, which, though fitful, wants to extend to all the benefits enjoyed at first by a few. It is an explosion that has behind it extraordinarily potent values, habits, and desires.

While it is always pleasant to find villains—the high pay of physicians, the profits of medical device manufacturers, the profligate wastefulness of the system are common, popular targets—my argument will be that these are not our ultimate problems though they are real and important. It is our deepest and most cherished values themselves that have brought us our most troubling problems and dilemmas. We take it to be a good thing that people now live longer and that medicine can bring an even longer life still. We take it to be a sign of hope, and vigor, and human triumph that we can have so much medical progress, that nature can be brought to heel. We believe it a badge of our moral vigor that we try to meet all individual needs, that we place that value at the top of our list of ethical aspirations. Yet it is precisely that combination of ideals that has led us to a dangerous irruption of costs, and a no less dangerous loss of moral direction.

Of course we must find a way to manage costs. But something more is required. The financial crisis facing the healthcare system provides a superb, if probably painful, occasion to ask some basic questions once again about health and human life. Where are we going? Where *should* we be going? We have tried for some years to treat the growing problems as technical, subject to bureaucratic fixes. That has not worked. We have tried also to think about the individual's right and entitlement to healthcare. That has not proved altogether illuminating. What we have not done is to examine the very goals and ideals of contemporary medicine and healthcare. We have assumed we know what that is all about, and that the only important questions turn on means, economic or moral, not on our chosen ends. The premise of this book is that we do not know what we are about, and that we are looking at the wrong questions. It is our ends we must examine.

I have before my mind's eye a future healthcare system that seeks not to constantly conquer all disease and extend all life, but which seeks instead to enhance the quality of life; which seeks not always to overcome the failings and decline of the body, but helps people better accept and cope with them; which tries to keep in view that health is a means to a decent life, not a value in its own right; which works to help society curb its appetite for ever higher quality and constant improvements in healthcare. It is a system that aims to intensify inward, seeking not the endless conquests of all new frontiers, but only those that promise a more coherent individual life within a more coherent societal life. Implosion must replace explosion.

Our toughest problem is not that of a need to ration health-care, though that will be necessary. It is that we have failed, in our understandable eagerness to vanquish illness and disability, to accept the implications of an insight available to all: We are bounded and finite beings, ineluctably subject to aging, decline, and death. We have tried to put that truth out of mind in designing a modern healthcare system, one that wants to con-quer all diseases and stay the hand of death. We can score some victories in that battle, but we cannot ultimately win it. Yet we have created a system that works with the conceit that we can, and we have devised a way of life to go with that system which hides from our eyes what we are about. It is our vision of health itself, and many of our cherished ideals, that must be changed.

## COPING WITH MEDICAL SUCCESS

Medicine and healthcare have, for one thing, entered a new stage of their history, one where the successes of medicine and not its failures are—in the way they interact with our values—the main source of our problems. That success has raised expecta-tions beyond a sustainable point, addicted the system to an unending search for new and usually expensive technological solutions (many of them occasioned by earlier technological solutions), and guaranteed marginal gains for ever higher costs. Scientific medicine once thought itself standing on an open frontier, cheap to prospect, easy to plow, and endlessly rich in its great reward—better health and longer lives. But that frontier is, and must be, forever ragged and ultimately unconquerable. It takes, ironically, money and success to discover fully this truth, and we are now doing so.

A consequence of this insight is that affluent nations must ration healthcare more firmly and sternly than poor nations. The rich must make choices that the poor do not have. A common view of rationing is that it is necessary only when there is an absolute shortage of some good and that nothing can be done to improve the situation. A crowded lifeboat with finite supplies is the popular image. A better image of rationing in our situation is that of the wealthy individual or corporation on the verge of bankruptcy, their liabilities beginning to exceed their assets. In many cases, one reason is inefficiency and sheer wastefulness. Addressing these problems is where most efforts to avoid bankruptcy begin. But a second reason is much more difficult to deal with: A whole way of life, previously free of any constraints, must be radically changed.

The deepest moral problems in the provision of decent healthcare are those of the relationship between health and individual happiness (or well-being) and between health and the common good. The working assumption behind biomedical research and its clinical application is that there is a direct correlation between better health, a longer life, and enhanced human happiness. But that correlation is by no means clear. The fact that many individuals crippled, burdened, or disabled by illness are able to adapt well enough to their lives is one piece of suggestive evidence. Something other than their health determines their happiness. Still another suggestive item is the long struggle that has been waged to determine when to stop life-saving medical treatment. A longer life is not necessarily a more tolerable life.

If the deepest part of the problem of healthcare is that of the relationship between health and human happiness, any meaningful proposed solution must be integrated into an understanding of a whole way of life. We can to some extent define "health" and suggest some minimal standards for achieving it, and we can say a few things about the conditions and meaning of human happiness. Yet such efforts, however imperative, will always have about them an air of generality and abstraction. They can only take on full meaning within the setting of actual societies, and be given flesh only as part of some coherent pattern of social meaning, behavior, and institutional practice. What we make of disease and illness, the meaning we attribute to them, is not fixed. That will be a function of the place we give them in our lives, the kind of significance assigned them by society, and the way we communally interpret suffering, disability, decline, and death.

The most potent social impact of medical advancement is the way it reshapes our notions of what it is to live a life. The prospect of a longer and healthier old age, for instance, leads us to think about that phase of life differently than did our ancestors. The greatest attraction of technological innovation is its promise of first breaking the barriers of natural, biological constraints and then moving on to a dismantling of the cultural attitudes and institutions designed to live within those barriers. The impact of effective contraception on ideas and ideals of family life and family size is a good example of that phenomenon. But that process, so ingrained now as part of the lore of desirable social change, is full of hazards. We must determine whether the new possibilities—always rosy and full of promised benefits—will actually be better than the old ways. If we decide that the answer to that question is yes, then the question is: What kinds of new institutions, and with them what new barriers, should be created? The centrality of health to human life, and the social and economic power of the healthcare system in our political and moral life, can only mean that we must devise a full way of life—attitudes, practices, expectations, mores—to go with, and to shape, our healthcare system and the values that underlie it.

I cannot pretend, or hope, to "devise a full way of life." That is something that can only emerge over time through our joint efforts, the fruit of reflection, practice, and experience. I can only try to outline what that way of life might in general look like, and how we might go about realizing it. I can suggest a direction and present a sketch, hoping it will be attractive enough to merit further exploration and pursuit.

Consider some questions that we, as a society, might ask but rarely do. What is the meaning of human health, and what is the source of that meaning? Where and how should health fit into our understanding of human life? What should medicine, and the science behind it, seek in the long run? What place and importance should be given to healthcare in managing our political and social systems? How much and what kind of illness is compatible with happiness and satisfaction in life? What kind of a life is it appropriate to expect medicine to help us achieve? What kind of medicine is best for a good society? What kind of society is best to deploy, and control, the power of medicine to shape and modify human life? How much and what kind of health does a society need in order to be a good society? What is a "good society" such that we can ask such questions?

## CAN WE FIND ANSWERS?

A common objection to questions of this kind is that they seem to admit of no final answers and are resistant to public consensus. That is not necessarily true, though the answers may be long in coming and only partially articulated. They are, in any case, central and vital. The impact of health upon our personal lives, the power of the healthcare system to influence almost every other aspect of our common life, and the economic implications of the way we provide it should force us to seek common answers. We rarely do. They intimidate us with their difficulty. They befuddle us in the absence of a shared language of morality and values. They offer the possibility of threatening our pluralistic peace. They get in the way of the pragmatic incrementalism preferred in the political arena. They are just plain trouble. They also happen to be the right and unavoidable questions.

Our understanding of health and illness, death and disease, will stem from our more general way of understanding the meaning and contours of our life within our society, our way of life as a whole. That understanding will in turn help at the political level to shape our convictions about our individual and collective entitlements to good health and healthcare: Who is to provide it, pay for it, and take responsibility for it? At still another level, the way we put those convictions into practice will finally be by means of various technical and bureaucratic arrangements. The healthcare debate in the United States has for the most part focused on the technical and the entitlement levels. They are, politically, the most accessible and familiar. One of my purposes, however, is to add the first and most basic level to the public debate, to see if a way can be devised to talk openly, meaningfully, and sensibly in the public arena about health as part of our way of life. That there is diminishing reason to believe we can cope with the problem solely at the other two levels alone gives greater urgency to that task.

There is a powerful tendency either to deny that there is a serious allocation and rationing problem or to evade the pain of difficult choices. The denial frequently takes the form of invoking some as-yet-unseen medical breakthrough to counter the massive growth of healthcare costs for the elderly or those suffering from some common diseases. More research, we are told, will save us. But there are no simple or inexpensive cures over the next horizon for cancer, heart disease, Alzheimer's, or stroke, those great killers and cripplers of the elderly and many younger people as well. The medical history of the human body, in any event, suggests that some other diseases will quickly come along to take their place even if we could dispose of them. Who had heard of AIDS a decade ago? If it is unlikely that there will be medical miracles to rescue us, it is just as unlikely that there will be bureaucratic miracles. There is a widespread belief that we can find some managerial fix, some wonderful incentive scheme to get doctors to use only proven treatments based on parsimonious diagnostic procedures, for instance. That belief is matched in fervor only by the hope that we can find some entitlement fix, some scheme that reduces government expenditures while leaving patients satisfied with their nicely calibrated out-of-pocket expenses. Those are forms of denial also. They can be combatted only by some hard work at the first level, that of our values and way of life. That is the key to everything else.

I come to the notion of a "way of life" with a particular conviction.[4] We will not, I believe, be able to work out the problems of our healthcare system unless we shift our priorities and bias from an individual-centered to a community-centered view of health and human welfare. We cannot and ought not give up a respect for individual needs and dignity, but we can place them within a social perspective and allow that to color our understanding. We can, for instance, ask as our first questions: How much and what kind of health do we need for the common good, and what will collectively and communally help and improve us as a society? At present we ordinarily begin by asking just what it is that individuals need for their good health; if there are communal concerns, they are put in a subordinate position. I want to reverse that priority—to begin with the communal needs and to put individual needs, rights, and interests in the subordinate position. It is the latter that must act as restraint upon the former, not the other way around as at present.

It is an approach that, among other things, can help throw into sharper relief the societal conditions that foster a greater emphasis upon illness prevention and health promotion, and upon the role that background conditions of life play in fostering good health. The deepest thrust of this approach, however, is to pursue the idea that we cannot solve the allocation problem without doing that which is most resisted—deciding what is good for us as a society, not just as individuals. What kind of health, pursued in what way, with what conception of the human good, will make ours a decent society?

There are two broad practical implications that I will develop out of a societal perspective. The first is that it can be used to justify a minimal level of healthcare guaranteed to all, but just what is guaranteed is to be determined by societal goals and resources rather than by individual needs or desires (though the two will often be identical). The second implication is that a guaranteed level of healthcare is only sensible financially, and only feasible politically, if there are firm limits to the individual demands that can be made for medical cures. The public interest, that is, requires both a baseline of decent healthcare for all and the setting of limits to the quest for cure; the two requirements cannot be separated. Joining them together in one conception will make possible an understanding of healthcare that seeks to eventually find, and live with, a sensible set of boundaries and limits and a coherent wholeness. The present system expands outwardly, so to speak; it must now turn inward, enhancing life, not always trying to save and extend it.

A sense of urgency is in order. Even if we succeed in guaranteeing some minimal level of care for all, and succeed in bringing greater coherence to the system, we will increasingly be faced with the need to pay for more and more of our healthcare out of our own pockets. If we do not learn how to curb our aspirations, we face a future of growing anger and disenchantment. We will think ourselves unfairly denied what is ours by right—ever-improved health—and blame our neighbor and our society, not our own unreasonable desires. That would be a sad mistake. It is ourselves we must change, those selves that have looked to medicine to deliver us from the burdens of a body that insists upon its mortality. We will not be so delivered. Our task is to know what to do about that truth.

The organizational plan of the book is as follows. In Chapters 2 and 3, I look at two ideals that have long animated the American healthcare system. One of them is that it is a plausible and worthy goal to attempt to meet all individual health needs, to seek a cure for all disease. The other is that the quest for this goal is an economically feasible one if only sufficient efficiency is brought to bear, an efficiency that can be enhanced by basic biomedical research and ways of providing healthcare that are more cost effective. I argue that the ideal of meeting the individual need for cure and the faith in efficiency as a way of making that possible are mistaken. It is not simply that they are impractical as goals, which is one way they are wrong. More fundamentally, they are goals that fail to take account of inherent human limitations. They thereby run the risk of deluding us as individuals about the possibilities of our lives, and of severely distorting a balanced pursuit of societal well-being. Our present system of healthcare is faulty, but not just because it is chaotic and poorly designed. It is faulty because it seeks the wrong ends.

Where Chapters 2 and 3 have as their purpose that of showing why our present system is flawed in its basic premises, Chapter 4 will begin the more constructive work of developing an alternative. The most important task there is to present a societal perspective on health, one that can provide a solid foundation for a way of life that will give a sensible and proper place to health in our common existence. To achieve this, we must try to determine appropriate goals and ends for the bio-medical enterprise in the context of an examination of what constitutes the human good—a formidable but imperative task. In Chapters 5, 6, and 7, I will spell out the practical policy implications of the broad perspective I am urging. Chapter 5 argues that we must, once again, give primacy to caring instead of curing in providing healthcare. Everyone, I contend, should have a minimally adequate level of caring, but he or she cannot and should not expect or demand that all individual needs for cure can be met. The demands for cure must be firmly limited. In Chapter 6, I propose a set of priorities to balance our aspirations for curative medicine to meet our individual needs, on the one hand, and our societal need to set limits, on the other hand. In Chapter 7, I suggest some ways of making the approach I have developed politically feasible. In Chapter 8, I will take up a difficult problem engendered by my proposals: How are we to distinguish between the rationing and societal limitation of healthcare and the wrongful taking of life? Must a society that gives up an unlimited pursuit of individual cure be one that is indifferent to the value of life? If it is necessary to limit health resources, would it not make sense to allow more people the right to active euthanasia and assisted suicide? In the final chapter, I will take a closing look at three values this book calls into question: the pursuit of unlimited medical progress, freedom of choice, and the common rejection of consensual values on the goals of health and life.

# CHAPTER 2

# ON THE RAGGED EDGE: NEEDS, ENDLESS NEEDS

Two powerful ideals have in recent decades dominated the provision of healthcare in the United States. The first is that of meeting individual health needs. The second is that of doing so in a way that is economically efficient. The emphasis upon individual need has long drawn from two sources, that of the moral traditions of medicine, directed toward individual patient welfare, and that of deep-seated American traditions, placing the good of the individual at the heart of national values. Efficiency as a value has somewhat shallower historical roots, but it has nonetheless long been part of American business and institutional beliefs that waste ought to be eliminated and maximum results obtained at the lowest possible cost. With the pressures of inflationary healthcare costs, the value of efficiency has become all the more pronounced. It is the driving force behind cost-containment efforts, and the spirit invoked in most recent proposals for universal health insurance. Taken together, meeting need and promoting efficiency generate a deep conviction: If the most efficacious medicine could be provided in the most efficient way, then the health needs of each and every individual could be met at an affordable price.

That is a wonderfully bracing, but mistaken, conviction. The ideal of meeting all individual need is neither possible as a reality nor plausible as a moral goal. No level of efficiency will overcome that impossibility. Medical progress has undone it as a feasible goal and competing social demands have undercut it as a meaningful goal. We will always have to live with unfinished medical progress, an always rough line dividing past success and present failure. Yet because of the persistence of an emphasis upon individual need, we have been left with an impossible task, that of solving the social problem of allocation—how we should distribute our collective resources—with ingredients that are private and individual. The evidence that it cannot be done is all around us and grows day by day. As I will contend in the next chapter, moreover, the goal of efficiency and effective cost containment cannot be achieved unless the moral goal of meeting individual need is changed; they have become intimately related. The widespread belief that we can all get all we need if only we deliver healthcare efficiently is hopelessly wrong, a deep and fundamental illusion. We will never get all we think we need as individuals and will have to settle for something less. But it is possible that, if we can alter our understanding of individual need, and place it within a more meaningful societal context, we may actually be better served than we are at present. Quite apart from its impossibility as an actual achievement, the ideal of meeting individual need does not even promise to serve the human good, either that of individuals or that of society. It leads us to reckless aspirations, and to an inability to separate hopeful desire and genuine necessity.

The need for good health seems, at first glance, a basic and simple need, one that can be free of unchecked aspiration. We need good health in order that our body might function well, allowing us to do what we want or must do. The singularity of good health has always been its invisibility. When all goes well with our body, we do not notice it, but when it is sick we can notice nothing else. We do at that point feel the press of desire. We want, desperately so, to regain our good health, to restore it to invisibility in order that we can get on with our life. But beyond that obvious case, why should desire have any place at all in the quest for health? In devising public policy, moreover, why could we not use the meeting of individual health needs as the simple goal, carefully sorting out and putting to one side what is nothing more than unreasonable desire?

The plain answer to those questions is that we have all but lost our way. We cannot separate health needs from health desires in our own lives, and neither can we devise a public policy that can adequately separate them. I am not referring only to the common escalation of what we want into what we need, though that will be a potent force here as elsewhere. The fundamental problem stems from uncertainty about the limits of our health potential. How long a life can we live, ought we want to live, or do we need to live? How much pain and suffering can and should we be ready to endure? How much disability can we survive, and how much fitness do we need? How much unhappiness is compatible with mental health? How much psychological stability do we require? Those are questions about the place, and extent, of health in our lives, and about the human needs that underlie our unending quest for better health. The uncertainty that such questions generate is well exploited by a technological progress whose basic purpose is ostensibly to help us meet our needs, but which in fact systematically blurs the line between need and desire. We have lost our way because we have defined our unlimited hopes to transcend our mortality as our needs, and we have created a medical enterprise that engineers the transformation.

At the heart of the public demand for good health is the insistence that life not be burdened with illness and that death be held at bay. That understandable desire has been rendered plausible by medical advances. Disease causes illness and death, and disease we now know can be conquered. What can be done ought to be done, and what began as desire ends as need. That redefined need becomes open-ended and insatiable, admitting of no boundaries. This is the transformation of health goals that lies at the root of our present problems. We cannot hope to manage the healthcare system, or our own aspirations, unless we learn how to control this transformation and the dynamic behind it.

It is a dynamic that embodies a vision of human possibility, one whose scope and elements are widely familiar if not always coherently expressed as a whole. Let me try to articulate that reigning vision. It consists of three major ingredients: a broad, limitless definition of health; a highly subjective notion of individual need, one captivated by the diversity of personal goals and desires; and a strong view of human rights, in particular the right of individuals to have access to adequate healthcare. It is a vision that sees health as an unbounded good, that allows the individual considerable leeway in defining, or inventing, his or her own health needs, and that allows one to make in principle as much demand on the help of fellow citizens—in the name of his or her rights and their obligations—as is required to meet those needs. It is a wonderful vision, but it is seriously flawed. It is collapsing under its own weight, and it will no longer suffice to provide the foundations for a healthcare system.

## A SOURCE OF TROUBLE: THE WHO DEFINITION OF HEALTH

While there is no single source of our present troubles, the 1947 World Health Organization (WHO) definition of health is a good candidate, providing the first ingredient, that of an open-ended understanding of the concept of health. WHO's definition came to embody the aspirations of the developed countries of the world: "Health is a state of complete physical, mental, and social well-being and not merely the absence of disease or infirmity." The emphasis on describing health in a positive way and as something that must be "complete" is its distinctive mark.[1]

The story behind that expansionary definition is instructive. The World Health Organization came into existence between 1946 and 1948 as one of the first activities of the United Nations. The animating spirit behind the formation of the WHO was the belief that the improvement of world health would make an important contribution to world peace. Health and peace were seen as inseparable. Just why this belief gained ground is not clear from the historical record of the WHO. A lack of world health has never been advanced as a serious cause of World War II. More to the point, perhaps, was the conviction that health was intimately related to economic and cultural welfare, and they in turn to world peace.

A number of memorandums submitted to a spring 1946 Technical Preparatory Committee meeting of the WHO capture the flavor of the period. The Yugoslavian memorandum noted that "health is a prerequisite to freedom from want, to social security and happiness." France stated that "there cannot be any material security, social security, or well-being for individuals or nations without health . . . the full responsibility of a free man can only be assumed by healthy individuals." The United States contended that "international cooperation . . . in . . . all matters pertaining to health will raise the standards of living, will pro- mote the freedom, the dignity, the happiness of all peoples of the world." But it was Dr. Brock Chisholm of Great Britain, soon to become the first director of the WHO, who personified what he called the "visionary" view of health. "The world," he argued, "is sick and the ills are due to the perversion of man: his inability to live with himself. The microbe is not the enemy: science is sufficiently advanced to cope with it were it not for the barriers of superstition. . . . The scope of the task before the Committee knows no bounds."

In Dr. Chisholm's statement are those elements of the WHO definition that gave it its power. It defined the problems of the world as a sickness, affirming that science would be sufficient to cope with the causes of physical disease, asserting that only anachronistic attitudes stood in the way of a cure of both physical and psychological ills, and declaring that the worthy cause of health can tolerate no limitations. It gave a powerful political and social mandate to the improvement of health, one that worked in tandem with the growing conviction that money invested in basic biomedical research would yield a powerful medical div- idend. The rapid postwar growth of the National Institutes of

Health in the United States, originally established in the late 1930s, was testimony to this belief. At the core of the WHO definition was a powerful though not self-evidently true conviction, that there is some intrinsic relationship between the good of the body and the good of the self, and between the good of the individual self and the good of the larger community, even the global community. For countries affluent enough to take it up, the basis was thereby laid for unlimited spending on health as a social good, and the health of the individual as the source of social good.

The WHO definition of health has never lacked its critics.[2] The most common charge has been that the very generality of the definition, and particularly its association of health and general well-being, has given rise to a variety of errors. Among them are the political tendency to define all social problems, from war to crime in the streets, as "health" problems; the blurring of lines of responsibility between and among the professions, and then between the medical profession and the political order; and the implicit denial of human freedom that results when failures to achieve social well-being are defined as forms of "sickness," somehow to be treated by medical means. The WHO definition replaced the traditional definition of health as bodily integrity and wholeness with a far more ambitious one, that of individual well-being more generally.

Despite these criticisms, the animating power of the definition has remained, sinking deeply into the bones of the American healthcare system and the political order that pays for it, and even more deeply perhaps in America than in many other countries also influenced by it. Given the possibility of endless medical progress, moreover, it is an almost inevitable definition, one implicit in the intellectual and ideological premises of the medical research enterprise itself. The WHO definition is at one with well-accepted, conventional ideas of medical progress. We need, therefore, to look more closely at it.

The most basic problem with the definition is that, by including the notion of "social well-being," it turns the enduring problem of human happiness and well-being into one more medical problem, to be dealt with by scientific means. It is a definition that finds (even as it creates) a fertile soil. How are human beings to achieve well-being or happiness? That is a fundamental question of life, and the WHO definition of health ties it closely to health. But is this self-evidently correct? Obviously illness, whether physical or mental, makes happiness more elusive, though not necessarily unattainable. There is no particular reason to believe that medicine can do anything more than make a modest, finite contribution to it, however important on occasion it can be in providing a necessary condition for the pursuit of happiness. Good health is, moreover, not even always a necessary condition of well-being. Illness does not preclude happiness or guarantee misery. Too obsessive a quest for health can, for that matter, also make it harder for people to achieve happiness. They can mistakenly believe that the answer to some of the great mysteries of live—love and death, joy and suffering—can be had through medical means. They are thus led down a dead-end road, the way paved with drugs and pills, tests and procedures—an endless pulse-taking to make certain that life goes on.

The WHO definition overturned many long-standing assumptions about medicine and health, especially its limited role in assuring general well-being. That was a mistake. Health is only a part of life, and the achievement of health only a part of the achievement of satisfaction with one's life. Medicine's role, however important, is limited. It can neither solve nor even cope with the great majority of social, political, and cultural problems; and it cannot even guarantee health. While it is good for human beings to be healthy, medicine is not morality. To be healthy and well is not necessarily to be a whole and full person. Medicine can save some lives, but it cannot be the most important institution in a society. Medicine can relieve much pain and some suffering, but it cannot relieve the ordinary burdens of living a human life or provide the general political or social conditions requisite for a flourishing common life.

Now that simply might be the end of the story, assuming some agreement can be reached that the expansionary impulse behind the WHO definition of health is an error. But I am left uncomfortable with such a flat, simple conclusion. The nagging point about the definition is that, in overstated ways, it was privy to the powerful insight that it is difficult to talk meaningfully of health solely as "the absence of disease or infirmity." What positive state of affairs are disease and infirmity an absence of? Against what are they being compared? The best we have historically been able to answer is to focus on the wholeness of the body, or its integrity.[3] Those terms suggest that good health represents the proper functioning, the correct harmony of the parts of the body, just the kind of functioning which gives the healthy body the kind of invisibility noted earlier. But those classical ideas have always implied a positive state of some kind, not merely the absence of some harmful conditions. The full pursuit of that issue if beyond the scope of this book, but it is necessary to bring to a discussion of health resources some substantive notion of health. What is it that we want to protect or enhance in the individual and distribute through the health-care system?

For the purpose of discussing allocation issues, we can usefully distinguish between health as a norm and health as an ideal. As a norm, it would be possible to speak in terms of deviation from some statistical standards, particularly if these standards were couched in terms not only of organic function but also of behavioral functioning. Thus someone can be called "healthy" if his heart, lungs, and kidneys function at a certain average level of efficiency and efficacy, if he can hear and see in a no less average way, if he is not suffering physical pain, and if his body is free of those pathological conditions that even if undetected or undetectable could impair organic function and eventually cause pain, illness, and death. When I go for a physical examination, my physician looks first for some deviation from accepted standards of average physical and biological functioning.

This way of thinking might be perfectly sufficient and satisfactory in a medically stagnant, or static, culture, and to a certain extent that is just the way we do think. The more subtle problem is that any notion of a statistical norm will be influenced by some kind of ideal of the self and its relationship to the body. Health presents itself as an ideal, a good, and not just a set of averages. Why should anyone care at all how his organs are functioning, much less how well they do so? Could it possibly be because certain departures from the statistical norm carry with them important implications for the self, for what the self considers good for it, an idea that transcends the medical state of the body? It would seem so. It is impossible, in fact, to draw any sharp distinction between conceptions of the human good— what benefits the self and its goals—and statistical norms of the body. This is the whole point of saying, in partial defense of the WHO definition of health, that it points to the intimate connection between the good of the body and the good of the self.

Are we not then forced to say, to push the issue a step further, that if the complete absence of health represented by death means the complete absence of self, then any diminishment of health must represent, correspondingly, a diminishment of self? Not at all. As the experience of many people shows, a strong, active self is consistent with a heavy burden of disease and disability. The self and the body are not, it turns out, quite one and the same—even if a severe toothache can sometimes do what a fatal cancer does not always do: dominate our sense of self to the point of utter distraction and despair. We are left, then, with a profound puzzle, that of the relationship between health and individual human happiness. To be happy is not necessarily to be healthy, and to be healthy is not necessarily to be happy. That is what the WHO definition, and its accompanying philosophy, failed to concede. That definition, while sensitive to an important truth about health, also embodied a view of the relationship between health and human well-being in general that is not simply wrong. When joined with the idea of meeting individual needs it also adds a burden to our thinking about health policy that is bound to increase demands for health beyond prudent boundaries, and even the pursuit of which takes us down a hazardous road. This will become evident when we look more closely at what it means to pursue the second ingredient of the reigning vision, that of meeting individual needs.

## DEFINING OUR NEEDS

Nothing would seem more appropriate as a goal of healthcare than the meeting of individual health needs. We want to live and not to die, to be well rather than to be ill. We do not invent those goals. They seem part of our nature, basic and necessary conditions of our existing and flourishing as human beings. To call them "needs" is nothing more than to say that, without them, we can neither be nor be ourselves. Yet there is something oddly elusive about the idea of a "need," even if we look carefully at the individual. We call something a need because, unless it is met, we cannot achieve our other goals; yet that means we can say little about the significance of the needs unless we can define those goals. How much and what kind of health we want depends in part on what we want to do with our life. This is particularly true if it is a question of how long a life we would hope for, or how much physical vigor we think necessary, or how essential psychological stability might be. Before long we are forced to ask some broad and difficult questions about human nature and our own destinies. What goals ought we to have as human beings? What kind of life should we live? What do we want to do with the life that good health can give us?

The idea of need becomes all the more elusive in a liberal, pluralistic society that believes it wrong for the society even to try to determine what goals and ultimate ends are appropriate for individuals, to say just what it is that we should as persons seek in our lives. The idea that there is, or could be, a good common to all people, a part of their nature, is usually rejected. It is a notion that seems to fly in the face of a commitment to individual choice and self-determination, and in the face of a widespread belief that no unitary human good has or will be discovered.[4] Technological progress plays into this cultural tendency by exploiting the desire for self-control and self-direction, and by the unwillingness and inability of the society to declare easily that the progress desired by some might pose a hazard, or burden, to others. But can we define "need" in some value-neutral way, and do so in a manner sufficiently solid to use it as the foundation for the allocation of healthcare?

To get at that question, it is first necessary to specify some meaning for individual "need" in the health context.[5] Three fundamental human needs can be identified, and they lend themselves to a health explication. The first need is simply to be, by which I mean to exist, to live. That is the necessary foundation for all other human activities and that is why laws against murder are the most primary in any society. The next need is to think and to feel. We are rational, emotional, and social animals. An inability to think will mean that we have no chance to understand and manage our situation in the world or to know what sense there is to be made of things. An inability to feel cuts us off not only from the depths of our own self, but also from the richness of relationships with others; we are, as Aristotle long ago noted, social beings. While thinking and feeling can conceptually be separated, they are ordinarily joined in our actual lives. The third need is to act, to be an agent that can do something in the world. It is action that most visibly takes us out of ourselves, that extends ourselves to others and to the world around us, that changes the world in which we live or enables us to adapt our behavior to a world we cannot change.

These three needs may be spelled out in a health context as follows. We have what I will call *body needs*, corresponding to the need to be, to exist. The good health of our bodily organs is a necessary condition for our being alive at all. While the capacities of those organs can be compromised, and some even dispensed with altogether, there is a minimal level below which we cannot fall without the threat of death. The priority typically given to the saving of life in healthcare expresses the importance of our body needs. Our need to think and to feel I will call our *psychological needs*. A failure to have those needs met will mean our diminishment as human beings. We will be unable to live with ourselves or to enter into relationships with others. A mental impairment, as in Alzheimer's disease, or an emotional crisis, as in depression, will leave us crippled as a self. Our need to act I will call our *function needs,* encompassing within that term all those activities that enable us to do something, either to perceive the world (vision and hearing, for example) or to act in the world (walking and speaking, for instance). The capacity for action, mobility, and perception allows us to manage and respond actively to the world around us.

Those definitions of needs can only be approximations, but they are sufficient to point us in a promising direction. We can then integrate into them some familiar categories of healthcare. We can distinguish between acute illness (posing an immediate and dire threat to one of our needs, e.g., appendicitis as a dire threat to our body needs or hallucinations as a threat to our psychological needs) and chronic illness (e.g., arthritis as a threat to our functional needs, or Alzheimer's disease). As Alzheimer's reminds us, some diseases will be threats both to our bodies and to our minds. Others, by contrast, will threaten our function needs (paraplegia) but leave other needs fully or partially capable of satisfaction—for the paraplegic can think and feel.

The possibility of many combinations and permutations here is one reason for the complexity of our health needs and of the resources required to meet them. The goal of medicine to help us meet our health needs is not so straightforward a task as it might at first appear. We can have some vital organs compromised and yet live on, our psychological resources intact. We can be depressed and, despite the good order of our organs, not desire to live at all. We can, if young and recently crippled by an athletic injury, prefer to die, putting the focus of our emphasis on our function needs and, even more narrowly, on our athletic aspirations. Or we can, if older and wiser, be relatively satisfied despite a life of immobility if we have our wits about us and our psychological needs met. I simply underscore here the great adaptability of human beings, on the one hand (survival and some degree of flourishing are possible while many needs are thwarted), and the great variability of human beings, on the other (life can seem empty when most, but not all, needs are being met, or if all needs are being met but not in ways that satisfy us).

As a first approximation, then, we can make some headway with the idea of human need. We can describe common features of our lives, root them in basic human needs, find their correlates in the realm of health, and then determine how to apply medical means to relieve any deficiencies. We can also make a distinction of great importance between *curative medicine* (designed to restore our body and its functioning to a state of normalcy in the face of illness, or to forestall a deterioration of capacity) and *caring medicine*, which I will define as providing social, psychological, and palliative support when cure cannot be effected (or afforded, as the case may be).[6] (I will us the term "the healthcare system" because it is a familiar one, even though it encompasses both curative and caring medicine.) That the permutations and combinations, the shadings and gradations, of needs can become complex should not in itself be an impediment to understanding. These complexities simply show us the breadth and richness necessary to pursue medicine and the healing arts. They begin to become a problem, however, when policy must be made and, in particular, allocation and rationing decisions are required.

Is a severe depression worse than chronic arthritis? Is a life-threatening heart attack more devastating than a drawn-out struggle with Alzheimer's? Is the loss of mobility worse than the loss of sight, or the loss of psychological stability as in paranoia worse than the inability to breathe well, as in emphysema? No one can provide a definitive answer to questions of that kind. Much depends, we will ordinarily say—on the person, on the circumstances, on the extent to which the suffering can be relieved—and that seems the right answer. But answers of that kind may not be good enough for policy purposes, where we are required to make some decisions, to set some social priorities. We may simply not be able to meet all those different needs equally. Then we must make some choices among them, as displayed in the 1987 Oregon decision to choose prenatal care over organ transplants (and its later efforts to devise a more comprehensive set of priorities).

Let me return to the original reigning vision here. That vision begins with a broad definition of health, presupposes that there are individual needs to be met, and that there is a societal obligation to meet them in some adequate way (or a right of individuals to have them met). The problem, however, is that two broad notions are being put together: a wide-ranging notion of health, and a no less wide-ranging notion of individual need. The policy issue then becomes acute when an effort is made to specify just what might count as an adequate, or minimum, or medically necessary level of curative medicine. Specific standards must be fashioned from expansive and open-ended generalities about health and individual need. A great additional obstacle is the widespread belief that in the end only individuals themselves can properly and adequately define their needs and that any fixed, government-imposed notion of the good of the individual should be denied.

It is revealing to see how difficult the task of fashioning standards of adequacy has been in the formation of policy. The issue can be put as follows. Let us agree that some degree of good health is necessary for human flourishing and to fulfill our individual needs. Let us also agree that some degree of access to healthcare is required to help us achieve it. What, then, might count as a baseline level of adequate level of healthcare, one that a society should seek to provide for everyone? A number of phrases and propositions have been developed to articulate this general idea. Among them have been that of a right to a "decent minimum" of care, or the meeting of "medical necessity" as a minimal standard of care to be guaranteed as part of the federal Medicaid program, or that of "basic care" as a way of summarizing the minimum package of subsidized care, or that of "normal species functioning" as a standard for the provision of care.[7] The phrase "adequate care" was used in a prominent report of the President's Commission for the Study of Ethical Problems in Medicine and Biomedical and Behavioral Research: "Society has a moral obligation to ensure that everyone has access to adequate care without being subject to excessive burdens."[8] While these phrases are not exactly equivalent, they all point to a similar concept: that some basic level of curative medicine necessary to meet a universal set of individual needs could be specified and then used for policy purposes. Even the President's Commission, while conceding the problems inherent in talking about needs, implicitly makes use of the concept.[9]

## THE MYTH OF ADEQUACY— NEEDS, ENDLESS NEEDS

Yet no sooner have such levels of curative medicine been specified than they run into immediate problems, particularly death by a thousand qualifications.[10] The standard of adequacy must not be so low that many legitimate individual needs would be excluded, or so high that it would require an unavailable or ridiculously high level of medical advancement and expenditures. Nor can it be a fixed and inflexible standard, good for all times and in all places; it must be relative to the resources and expectations of different societies. One common solution to difficulties of this kind—that of the inescapability of endless qualifications and disagreements about needs—is to leave determinations of "minimum," "necessary," and "adequate" to the political process.[11] Do not define them, simply let people vote their own meanings and preferences. But even if that is not already a counsel of despair at making sense of the idea of a "minimum" or what counts as "adequate," how are voters themselves supposed to find a sensible position for which to vote? What are they supposed to think about? To make the problem one of pure political process may be nothing more than a way of evading the problem under the guise of dealing with it. Voters will have the same problem as experts. They will not know what might count as a sensible standard.

The breakdown of kidney dialysis selection committees in the late 1960s, prior to Medicare coverage of dialysis, perfectly illustrates the problem. Mixed committees of laypersons and medical people were asked to decide which patients—based on unspecified personal, familial, and social criteria—should be allowed access to dialysis machines, then in short supply. The committees literally had to make life-and-death decisions. They reported themselves unable to make meaningful comparisons and choices. They could not devise appropriate moral criteria either. They considered their effort a failure.[12] The same experience, now writ large, is likely if the political process is left to make the decision but given no moral standards to help guide it.

There is another important, and overlooked, consequence of the difficulty in defining individual needs. In recent years hope has been placed in a number of quantitative techniques meant to aid the decision-making process in allocation dilemmas. Almost all, in some way, seek to maximize a specified goal (longevity, or effective cure, or relief of pain, for instance) and to arrive at a balance of some greater good. Cost-benefit analysis, the most common of these techniques, seeks to determine how to balance the cost of a treatment against its likely benefits. But the notion of a "benefit" often proves elusive, precisely because individuals will specify their needs in different ways and there is too little societal consensus on the value of having different needs met; the concept of "benefits" is rarely quantifiable.[13] The same kind of problem befalls QALYS—"quality adjusted life years."[14] Here the goal is to determine which medical expenditures will most maximize a combination of the quality of life and the length of life. But there is no agreement on what the proper ratio is, and thus no effective way to use the technique to make decisions across populations that may differ in their assessment of what it means to have their needs met.

What are we to make of the general failure to find a feasible and adequate way of giving content to the idea of meeting individual needs? Is it just an accident that all efforts to find meaningful definitions of "adequate" or "minimal" or "necessary" have failed? Is it from a lack of sufficient effort that they all turn out to be either too general to be of any practical use or too much a shopping list of diverse needs to constitute a coherent or meaningful whole? The failure, I believe, is inevitable, inherent in the project itself. Part of the problem reflects the standard difficulties of agreeing on anything about individual lives in pluralistic societies: Class, education, ethnicity, income, and the like characteristically lead people to develop different notions of what they aspire to and want, what they think they need, and what they will settle for. Thus on those grounds alone we should expect trouble.

That trouble deepens when we must make allocation decisions. We can agree on the value of setting a broken leg, but when we have to decide whether to invest in a neonatal care unit, or an expensive drug benefitting a few for a short time only (AZT for the treatment of AIDS), or bypass surgery for octogenarians, or expensive rehabilitation for auto accident victims, then consensus collapses. At that juncture, the combination of varying individual needs, the expression of different wants and desires, the resistance to imposed solutions, and the pressure of competing societal needs renders the use of "need" as a standard all but useless. David Braybrooke, in a book that is an otherwise powerful defense of the concept of "need" as a viable one for policy purposes, concludes that "nothing . . . in the concept of needs saves the need for medical care from becoming a bottomless pit."[15]

## MEDICAL PROGRESS AND INDIVIDUAL NEED

More fundamentally, however, it is medical progress itself that has rendered the enterprise of defining individual curative need as impossible, and thus with it notions of finding some identifiable baseline of healthcare to be provided to all. That progress has created three insuperable obstacles to defining "minimal" needs or "adequate" care: (a) denying the limits of the possible; (b) widening the gap between individual needs; and (c) systematically blurring the line between desire and need by raising expectations and permitting individual choice of goals and quality of life.

# Denial of the Limits of the Possible

Consider the need of the body to live. What can medicine bring to that need? It has already brought vaccines and antibiotics to deal with lethal infectious disease, respirators and dialysis units to cope with failing organ systems, transplants to provide new organs, surgery to remove tumors and repair lesions, and general biological knowledge to help us prevent potentially fatal disease. How far can all of this go? Who knows? There are no known theoretical limits. Mortality from heart disease has fallen in recent decades and continues to decline, and while cancer has yet to be conquered, there is no reason not to expect continuing progress. Organ transplantation becomes gradually more successful, and while there is a limit because of the availability of organs for transplant purposes, there is no necessary limit to the possibility of artificial organs. A gradual sharpening of the distinction between growing old (which cannot be helped) and becoming sick (which can be dealt with) does not make old age as such (in the eyes of some, at any rate) a necessarily fatal condition. Our need to live, then, admits of no discernible medical boundaries. There is no individual medical condition that does not, in principle, admit of the possibility of an eventual cure or significant amelioration. The most desperate class of patients, with the rarest of diseases, may eventually have their need to live met. It cannot be ruled out. Even now, available medical techniques can be used to gain a few hours, or days, even in the most desperate cases (which is one reason the termination of treatment has proved so difficult even with obviously dying patients).

To make these observations is to say more than that the standards of what counts as minimal or adequate will change over time. It is to say at least that much, but it is also to say that even at any given time it will not be possible to specify the necessary standards except in relatively arbitrary ways. There will be, for one thing, the claims of interest groups for resources to cope with the disease or condition of concern to them. Their aim is to *change* the existing standards, to declare them inadequate right now, to exploit research and clinical possibilities, and to expand our notions of the possible and desirable. There will, for another, be the claims of critically ill individual patients. It will be almost impossible in many cases to say that a patient could not, in some way, benefit from further efforts, or from a different method of treatment—his or her need might yet be met; something, however experimental, might already be available. Most important, one suggested and valuable standard, that of "normal species functioning," can readily be thrown into doubt.[16] We know neither, at the upper end, just what we might aim for—how good our health might be, or how long our life might be—nor, at the lower end, what deprived level of functioning is (with technological assistance) minimally compatible with a satisfactory life.

The term "normal" comes to lose all meaning in the face of constant medical progress, whose very purpose, in its most ambitious moments, is to redefine "normal," to give us a new picture of human possibility. Our need to live, for instance, admits of no necessary boundary, either in our individual case or in the case of groups or classes of people afflicted with otherwise fatal illnesses. Why should we accept a now-normal average life expectancy of seventy-five years if medical science could give us something better? Is not the history of medical advancement one of running roughshod over supposedly immutable ideas of normalcy?

Or consider our psychological needs. The enormous expansion of demand for mental health services in recent years reflects a widespread belief that psychological needs can be as important as physical needs, and that therapy to meet psychological needs can be as helpful, even decisive, as therapy to meet physical needs.[17] Both the research trend toward seeking a biological basis for the most serious pathologies (schizophrenia and depression, for instance) and the therapeutic trend toward short-term psychotherapies for lesser problems promise a growing ability to provide some help to most people, either now or at least in the future. The need for counseling and therapeutic help itself steadily expands, and the range of problems dealt with continues to widen, now encompassing substance abuse. This expansion is driven by a public perception of emotional and mental problems as now more socially acceptable than in the past, by the inclusion of therapy for them as part of standard packages of healthcare, and by the belief that such therapy can be efficacious. While there has been considerably less progress with the major and minor tranquilizers, as well as other psychoactive drugs, than was earlier thought possible, there remains a strong sense of optimism that the advances will eventually emerge. There is, then, no discernible boundary to what people will come to define as a psychological need and to what the various health sciences can do to respond to that need.

Last, consider the need to function. At one time, the fate of someone who had suffered a devastating accident and came out of it as a paraplegic or quadriplegic was grim. A short and cruel life was likely. Now rehabilitation has progressed. The infections that would have carried him off earlier can now be controlled, and skilled rehabilitation making use of technological devices can give him the possibility of some eventual mobility. Even more can be done for the elderly stroke victim. He or she can now be helped to regain speech and the use of paralyzed arms or legs, and can often enough be restored to normalcy. A gradual improvement in hearing aids deals with a less critical malady, but one that is important and widespread among the elderly. The severely handicapped newborn can be provided with shunts to drain excess fluid in the brain, artificial assistance for malfunctioning kidneys, surgery for a defective heart, and transplants for failed organs. Improved fetal surgery will eventually be able to correct some conditions prior to birth. The gradual rejection of the term "vegetable" applied to any human being reflects not simply repugnance at the use of a demeaning term. It also signals the growing optimism that hardly any human being, no matter how handicapped of disabled, is beyond some rehabilitation.

A denial of the limits of the possible in effecting cures is thus a central part of the ideology of scientific medicine. It is sustained in part by its actual success in overcoming earlier obstacles and curing illnesses once thought beyond reach, and in part as an act of faith that is at one with the general faith in science. But it is a most potent faith, reaffirmed again and again by actual advances.

## Widening of the Distance between Individual Needs—Creating Vertical Gaps

If it is a part of the reigning idea of medical progress that there are no fixed limits to the therapeutic possibility of cure of amelioration, and thus no boundaries to the meeting of individual needs, that same progress widens the gap among individuals in their potential demand on the healthcare system. One person, the most lucky, may only require a shot of penicillin at a cost of a few dollars to deal with a minor infection over the course of a lifetime—and the healthcare system can meet his individual need. Another person, not so lucky, may require a kidney transplant at a cost of over $200,000 to save his life, and still others may over the course of an extended illness require treatment costing as much as $1.5 million to $2 million; their needs, with more difficulty, might also be met. One newborn child may require a few extra days in the hospital for a few thousand dollars to clear up a minor problem while another may need months in a neonatal intensive care unit at a cost of over $400,000 (and perhaps additional years of extended rehabilitation once discharged); still another may require $800,000 worth of care. The possibilities of expensive rehabilitation for the teenage motorcycle victim or the elderly sufferer of a stroke—possibilities developed only recently—to mention other examples, are enormous. The chaos of state or county healthcare budgets devastated by highly expensive treatments needed by a handful of patients has become a not-uncommon story. A $2 million child welfare budget for an entire county consumed by only a few patients requiring extended neonatal care poses nearly impossible dilemmas for the officials who must manage such budgets. The only perfect escape is a constantly escalating budget, one designed to keep up with medical progress.

These commonplace instances point to what I would call the increasing *vertical gap* of care, that is, the widening cost of curative and life-saving care between the least and most expensive patients, both with the same and with different conditions. That vertical gap can take different forms. One is the gap between different patients with the same condition, a simple versus a complicated newborn case where both are, say, the result of a premature birth. Another is the gap between those with common, inexpensively treated conditions (pneumonia, for instance) and those with rare, expensively treated conditions (major organ failure). Still another is between those with common diseases for which cures (expensive or inexpensive) already exist and those with diseases that are both rare and as yet untreatable, but which might be treatable after more research. There may be what the economists call "marginal returns" in investments designed to equalize treatment for those who experience the gap, but it may just as well be that, if enough money is invested, the return for closing the gap could be a good one. But the cost of trying to do so may be enormously high.

The problem of the vertical gap is a direct consequence of attempting to meet individual needs. Those needs are diverse, but the progress of medicine is being able to do so with a widening range of patients means that there are also few boundaries here. Where death or illness would once quickly have taken the lives of those who suffered severe accidents or illnesses, they can now often be saved; but many can be saved only at great cost. Earlier, the costs would have clustered within a moderate range; now they can wildly vary. Yet if the accepted goal is the meeting if individual curative need—to give everyone a chance at, say, "normal species functioning"—then there is no logical choice but to accept the widening, and necessarily widening, vertical gap. By virtue of redefining what is "normal" and having more success at the margin, the possibilities of pursuing individual need become unlimited. It is just such situations, of course, that have occasioned a hope in cost-benefit analysis. But precisely because there is no way to quantify, or morally judge, the comparative benefits of meeting quite different individual needs, the technique must fail.

The possibilities have rarely been put better than they were by Enoch Powell, during his tenure as minister of health in Great Britain: "There is virtually no limit to the amount of medical care an individual is capable of absorbing. . . . Not only is the range of treatable conditions huge and rapidly growing, there is also a vast range of quality in the treatment of these conditions. . . . There is hardly a type of condition from the most trivial to the gravest which is not susceptible of alternative conditions affording a wide range of skill, care, comfort, privacy, efficiency, and so on. [Finally] there is the multiplier effect of successful medical treatment. Improvement in expectation of survival results in lives that demand further medical care. The poorer (medically speaking) the quality of the lives preserved by advancing medical science, the more intense are the demands they continue to make."[18]

## Blurring the Line between Aspiration and Need

Medical progress has meant the near-banishment of fatalism. Given enough time, money, scientific research, and clinical ingenuity—it is widely believed—no disease, no disability, no stressful psychological state is beyond cure or amelioration. Our aspirations and hopes are at first made credible by medical progress; then, as they move closer to realization, they come to have the status, and the insistence, ordinarily accorded to need. This is the transformation of desire or aspiration into putative need. No one thought, a century ago, that a person suffering from heart disease "needed" a heart transplant; death was simply accepted. But the advent of heart transplants was stimulated first by hope, and that hope became concrete need as transplantation succeeded. People now "need" heart transplants. A whole new category of need has been created, a need orginally thought to encompass only younger people but now coming to include older patients as well.[19]

More and more people can be cured of their illnesses, and thus more aspirations turned into needs, those who cannot be cured can be better maintained or rehabilitated, and those who can only be maintained can be given an improved quality of life. That is the faith of modern medicine. When that deeply rooted faith is combined with the high value given individual choice and self-determination, then the meeting of individual need has still another dimension added to it. It will be left to the individual to decide what constitutes need and a decent "quality of life." That the idea of individual quality of life is notoriously subjective is one reason to leave it to individual choice. Still another is that, in a liberal society, it is taken as inappropriate to set societal standards about individual desires and needs. That would require a substantive and deep view of what is ultimately good for individuals, what they should find life worth living for, or be willing to live with. The irony, of course, is that by refusing to repudiate individualist conceptions of need, costs climb so damagingly high that the individual eventually loses. A paradoxical tyranny of egalitarianism also emerges. As we find more complex and expensive ways of meeting individual need, the demand rises that all should have access to such treatments; we then push on, creating still another crisis of equality with further medical progress. Yet we continue to bless the meeting of individual need.

The consequences of this widespread view can only be the blurring of the line between desire and need, particularly when combined with a belief in the indefinite possibility of medical progress. There is, above all, the problem of rising expectations, which opens the distance between aspiration for health and its actual achievement. As Dr. Arthur J. Barsky has shown with solid statistics, the actual improvement of health over recent decades has not been matched by a subjective sense of better health. Not only do people "report more frequent and longer-lasting episodes of serious, acute illness now than they did 60 years ago . . . [there is also] a progressive decline in our threshold and tolerance for mild disorders and isolated symptoms, along with a greater inclination to view uncomfortable symptoms as pathologic—as signs of disease. . . . The standard we use for judging our health appears to have been raised, so that we are more aware of—and more disturbed by—symptoms and impairments that previously we deemed less important."[20] Barsky also notes that a focus on health promotion stimulates greater attention to the body and enhanced nervousness about its condition; that can occasion still more visits to a physician. The growing acceptability of the sick role and better insurance coverage to support it also enhance a heightened social tolerance of illness and medical intervention.

One is reminded here of a common problem of the rich, where increased wealth brings increased desire and expectation, yet an increase that is never satisfied, never sufficient. "A great deal of money, says [Malcolm] Forbes, allows you 'more of what you enjoy than you may need.' But needs have a funny habit of adjusting themselves: as one earns more, the bell curve of well-being, with a barely perceptible groan, shifts upward."[21] A comparable phenomenon in healthcare deserves the most careful reflection. At the least, it suggests that our felt state of satisfaction may bear little relationship to the way we actually are. Does that mean that one role for medicine to play is that of helping us to accept, and learn to cope with, our illnesses and disabilities? Yes, for medicine should not create unrealistic expectations, or stimulate ever-escalating desires. There is little, if any, reason to believe that the quest for endless medical progress will deliver correspondingly endless improvement in our sense of personal satisfaction with our health, much less with our life more generally.

Despite such considerations, nonetheless, we see the relentless and pervasive power of a desire for improved health. The lure of medical progress has so far proved too strong to be deterred by the absence of parallel happiness. It is, moreover, but a small step from increased expectations of progress for individuals to declare that their desires have the status of needs, and to use political pressure to make the healthcare system accept that transformation (as has happened with the category of mild mental disturbances, or the movement for the rights of the disabled). It is no less open to individuals to desire to extend the limits of their needs beyond earlier borderlines. If I want to live to be 100, well beyond present average life expectancy, why can I not define my failing organs as needy of life and maintenance (which they surely are in one sense) and demand of the healthcare system that it respect my free choice? If there are no "official" state views on what constitutes an acceptably long biographical or biological life, I am well within my rights to make my own choice on that matter; well within the bounds of reasonable expectation to think that medicine might be able to give me that life; and no less within my rights to demand that the healthcare system take account of my individual desire in this respect, a desire that is, after all, a need to stay alive, as basic a need as there is.

However we might best understand the informal logic of the transformation of desire into need, one fact seems indisputable. Healthcare expenditures rise in direct proportion to an increase in the gross national product, in the United States and elsewhere as well, but in a way much closer to the rising consumption of luxury items than to anything else. It has been observed, for instance, that there is an increase in caloric intake when there is an increase in the GNP. The ratio of that increase has been in the range of 1.5 to 1. Yet the corresponding ratio of increase in medical-care expenditures per capita has been 6 to 1, virtually the same ratio as the increase in consumption of fine wines and foreign travel. This suggests both the expansive power of health "needs" when money is available and the way in which desire can transform itself into need when money makes that possible.[22]

The line between need and desire or aspiration is, therefore, not only increasingly in principle indistinguishable, but it seems clearly the case that the best way to stimulate more desire is to meet real needs. That makes certain that the desires not yet met will be defined as needs still to be met—and so on, infinitely. Desires beget needs, and needs met beget further needs. As long as we want to live and to be other than what we are, it is hard—given the idea of medical progress—to see how matters could be otherwise.

## MEETING NEED: A RIGHT TO HEALTHCARE? __

Let me turn to the third part of the reigning vision. The idea of a right to healthcare, though often battered and rejected, remains a powerful one in American life. While it sometimes takes different forms—the right of access to healthcare, or the right to a decent minimum of care—central to the notion is that the individual has a legitimate claim of access to decent healthcare regardless of an ability to pay for it. If there is a right to life, many have argued, then a right to healthcare is its political implication.[23] Health, so the argument continues, is necessary to life, and without health the pursuit of other goods and other rights is rendered impossible or severely compromised. The focal point of the right to healthcare in its most common formulations is that of individual need.

The right to healthcare may be defined as a legitimate claim of the individual on society to have his or her health needs met. As the Universal Declaration of Human Rights has put it, "Everyone has a right to a standard of living adequate for the health and well-being of himself and his family, including food, clothing, housing, medical care and necessary family services."[24] Or, phrased differently by the American Medical Association: "It is the basic right of every citizen to have available to him adequate medical care."[25] Or, in a way that brings out the importance of health in relationship to other goods: "No one can fully, if at all, enjoy any right that is supposedly protected by society if he or she lacks the essentials for a reasonably healthy and active life. . . . Any fatal deficiencies end all possibility of the enjoyment of rights as firmly as arbitrary execution."[26]

Why has this claim, so powerful in the 1960s and 1970s, wavered in recent years, and why is there now reason to doubt it? Part of the reason is a proliferation of claimed rights in the name of individual welfare.[27] That has overloaded the concept of rights to the point of meaninglessness, creating a hopelessly complex array of competing rights. For some, it has seemed preferable (at least politically) to shift to the language of government obligation to provide care, and away from a claim of the individual to a right to healthcare. That is what the President's Commission did when it spoke of "a moral obligation to ensure that everyone has adequate care." Yet to talk of a societal obligation to everyone raises exactly the same kinds of problems in meeting individual need as does the language of rights (even though it may shift the political rhetoric in more tolerable ways).[28] How do we determine the nature and extent of the obligation to individuals?

I will put to one side the question of the preferability of the language of obligation over that of rights. We might instead stay with the claim of a right to healthcare and ask one question: What does is mean to pursue a "right to healthcare" in the context of medical progress and its impact on the idea of individual need and, most specifically, to pursue the right to curative healthcare? My answer is direct: The quest becomes an impossible one, doomed to frustration. The claim that we have a right to healthcare is a claim that our neighbor (ordinarily through the instrumentality of government) has an obligation to provide that assistance necessary to meet our individual health needs. But medical progress, far from clarifying those needs, renders them all the more problematical. If those needs do not admit, in principle, of any limits or any clear specifications, then there are no boundaries to our claim for healthcare, certainly none intrinsic to the concept of individual need itself. Since we have, moreover, allowed the value of choice and freedom to overshadow other considerations, we have relinquished the possibility of meaningfully distinguishing morally among needs or attaching any fixed priorities to them. The claim of a right to healthcare becomes, therefore, hopelessly vague and open-ended. It cannot be used to deny on its intrinsic merits anything claimed by the individual in the name of health nor, in the face of a plethora of claims, does it have the ethical resources to set priorities among them.

Limits to claimed rights can of course be set, but that must be done externally; that is, by bringing in considerations foreign to the centrality given the individual in the traditions both of medicine and of individual rights. Overriding economic needs and other social and political priorities are of course prime instances of such foreign intrusions. But the rational foundation for doing so in any way other than through the arbitrary force of political decisions has been destroyed. The struggle within the political process determines the outcome, based on expressed preferences and not necessarily on deeply grounded need. There is no unitary set of values, or goals, that guides the process.

What is the result? By making individual needs open-ended, and embedding those needs within the values of a liberal and pluralistic society, the possibility of order, coherence, and meaningful purpose has been lost. Interest groups have a powerful sway in this setting. They can pursue their own ends unimpeded by any larger design of healthcare goals or priorities. They do not have either to take into consideration the needs of other groups or to propose limits on their own demands. Why should they? There is no incentive, much less reward, for doing so. Their needs are, simply as needs, as important as anyone else's. Since we would not ordinarily think of a claimed need, say, to discover a cure for cancer as narrowly of pejoratively "self-interested," we are not prone to object to such campaigns (unless they seem wasteful and inefficient—the only effective charge that can be entered against them). The net result of many competing health interest groups, however, is that victory tends to go to those with the most political power or the most potent emotional claims. Many other important social needs can thereby be neglected, and there is no reason to think that the general level of health will necessarily be improved.

There is an even more deleterious impact in tying together the idea of rights and individual health needs. Because medical progress renders individual need open-ended and subject to no intrinsic limiting principle, we are left bereft of any clear notion of what kind and scope of healthcare we actually owe each other as a society. We can give no clear meaning to terms such as "adequate care" or "minimal needs," and thus cannot establish policy in any sound way. It is not for nothing that the lesson of the dialysis experience has stuck in the craw of Congress. Established in 1973 as a universal entitlement for all who require dialysis to save their lives from kidney failure—as clear a body need as one could ask—the program grew wildly beyond all early projections and encompassed a wider and wider group of users, some 80,000 at present, including about 30 percent over the age of sixty-five (and the fastest-growing group on dialysis, increasing on average by 13 percent a year).[29]

There has proved to be no feasible way to limit claims upon that program, however sick, old, or unpromising someone might be as a candidate for it. That is the direct and inevitable outcome of making individual need the criterion for access. Moreover, when surveyed, those on dialysis would prefer to continue dialysis even at the price of a great loss of quality of life; hence, medical efficacy itself is not necessarily the only measure of its acceptability to recipients. The widespread assumption that people would prefer to be dead than live a life of very low quality may be wrong. As the author of a study of kidney dialysis concluded, "We may no longer be able to take refuge in the belief that we are only prolonging misery. And if we conclude that the preference to live with an expensive, apparently debilitating chronic illness rather than die is reasonable, then we cannot, at the same time, expect to contain medical costs."[30] If the patient or the patient's physician wants it, he or she will get it. The patient determines need, and the patient determines what counts as a decent quality of life on dialysis. A consequent result is a trend for older and sicker patients to be on dialysis.[31] The fiscally terrifying prospect of similar results with all other illnesses by enacting additional unlimited entitlement programs, much less a comprehensive national health insurance program, has been a powerful obstacle to congressional action.

In that context, the slogan of a "right to healthcare" is one that rightly intimidates legislators. They know that such a claim, combined with intractable individual needs and constant medical innovation, could and probably must turn into an economic monster. The principle of a right to healthcare, lacking intrinsic limits, fails a most important contemporary legislative goal, that of developing principles of entitlement that contain within them some self-limiting boundaries. A principle that provides no way—as part of the principle itself—of setting priorities, no way of setting limits, and no way of setting shared societal goals cannot effectively be used for purposes of public policy. It is to write a blank check, to be filled in as each individual chooses and as medical progress conditions the individual to choose.

If there was some way of determining basic curative health needs, based on a commonly held substantive view of individual human good, that would provide us with the basis for devising a meaningful right to healthcare based on abiding human need. But since medical progress has already carried us well along the continuum of improved health, we both lack such a view of individual medical need at present and are unlikely to discover it in the future. At the same time, we have culturally accepted a notion of medical progress that makes it impossible to know where we should even look.

Does this conclusion require that the idea of individual need, particularly curative need, be eliminated altogether? That would be neither possible nor necessary. But it does show the necessity for a radically altered conception of need, one that is feasible of achievement and capable of being afforded. The curative needs of the individual simply as isolated individual cannot any longer be the dominating, much less exclusive, focus of the healthcare system. To the extent that a claimed right to healthcare (or obligation to provide healthcare) is solely oriented to meeting individual need, it must fail as well. But that principle does not necessarily preclude the possibility of finding a different moral basis for providing healthcare than individual curative need alone, and different moral foundation than that of individual rights (or societal obligation to the individual). It actually makes that task all the more urgent, because it has been a relentless holding on to that idea that has made our economic situation worse while at the same time failing to meet otherwise legitimate health demands. The widespread moral belief that the provision of healthcare must in some way be understood as a societal obligation and task requires a better moral foundation. That foundation must be, I will argue in Chapter 4, a societal, not individual, foundation.

To challenge the idea of meeting individual curative need (and to suggest limits to society's obligation to meet such needs) is no less than to question some fundamental features of our entire way of life. It is to question not its failures but what are thought to be its highest ideals. It is to challenge our belief in the possibility, and virtue, of unlimited medical progress. It is to challenge the centrality we have given to the individual and his or her personal needs. It is to challenge the view that there is a special societal obligation (generating a claim on our part) to meet our individual health needs, however deep and infinite those needs turn out to be.

For many, a challenge of this kind to the idea of a "right to healthcare" would seem a threat to decades of work to effect reform of a chaotic and unjust system. Is it wise to provoke challenges to such long-standing ideals? I do so only because those ideals are failing, and must fail. It is not that they were necessarily and obviously wrong from the outset. That would have been difficult to determine without some extended experience in pursuing and living with them. But we now have that experience, and we should have the nerve to take seriously what it is telling us. It is saying that the reigning vision I have tried to characterize—that of meeting individual need within a framework of an open-ended notion of health and medical advancement—cannot be sustained, that it rests on faulty premises. They are faulty premises about the benefits of unlimited medical progress, about what makes people happy and satisfied, and about what serves the common good of society.

Our continuing failure to find a meaningful way to define such phrases as "minimally adequate" and "medical necessity" should have alerted us that something was fundamentally amiss. We failed to see that they cannot be defined in any ultimately satisfactory way. That should now be clear. Our way of life as a whole has assumed the necessity of constant progress as the way to human happiness and well-being. We have simply incorporated our thinking about health into that context. It is a way of life that has denied the need for limits. A change in the way we think about health requires a change in the way we think about the living of a life.

## ON THE RAGGED EDGE: CARING AND CURING

Our main task as individuals, and as a society, will be to learn how to accept, and live with, what I will call the "ragged edge" of medical treatment and progress. Imagine that you are trying to tear a piece of rough cloth and want to do so in a way that leaves a smooth edge. Yet no matter how carefully you tear the cloth, or where you tear it, there is always a ragged edge. It is the roughness of the material itself that guarantees the same result; a smooth edge is impossible. No matter how far we push the frontiers of medical progress we are always left with a ragged edge—with poor outcomes, with cases as bad as those we have succeeded in curing, with the inexorable decline of the body however much we seem to have arrested the process. Whether it be intensive care for the premature newborn, low-birthweight baby, or bypass surgery for the very old, or AZT therapy for AIDS patients, the eventual outcome will not likely be good; and when, eventually, those problems are solved there will then be others to take their place. That is the ragged edge of medical progress, as much a part of that progress as its success.

The most vexing problem is not just that there is a ragged edge, however. There is bound always to be one if we are genuinely on the frontier. The inevitability of a ragged edge also makes it impossible to meet individual needs at the frontier; and individual health needs will *always* have their frontiers, most fundamentally our need to live on if we can do so. There will always be the possibility of improving the outcome with 500-gram babies (the present frontier of viability), or ninety-five-year-old patients suffering from multi-organ failure, or the quadriplegic teenage victims of auto accidents. We thus remain dissatisfied because it is the problems of those frontiers, on those ragged edges, that capture our attention and imagination. No matter how much progress we have already made, it is the progress we have not yet achieved that galvanizes the research and clinical community. That is where the death, pain, and suffering are now located.

The offices of doctors will always be full, no matter how much progress is made. There will always be those on the edge of that progress—an office full of different patients than, say, a century ago, but still, and always, a full office. There will always be death, pain, and suffering, and there will always be a medical frontier. Fifty years ago the frontier was elsewhere. By virtue of earlier progress, however, we have raised our hopes and expectations about future progress. Why should we settle for anything less than continuing progress on this year's frontier? For most people that would be a rhetorical question, particularly if it is they, or their loved ones, who are on the frontier (or the researchers interested, as always, in the frontier conditions). The ragged edge of the frontier, moreover, has two features in medicine: the failures (most common), and the occasional successes (the rare 500-gram baby who survives and flourishes). The failures elicit our empathy, goading us forward. The successes encourage us to keep going in the face of the failures. The combination of great failure at the edge and some success is a powerful one, ever pulling us onward.

Yet the point, of course, is that we cannot win the struggle with the ragged edge. We can only move the edge somewhere else, where it will once again tear roughly, and again and again. If this is so, and if the effort to defeat the ragged edge assures ever-rising costs (for many of the easier, cleaner tears were made earlier in history), when will we know when and how to stop? Not when and how to stop because further progress cannot be made—further progress can *always* be made; we have no reason to disbelieve that. But knowing how and when to stop because further progress entails either too great an economic or social price or too little likely improvement in the human condition, or both, is a far harder decision. Yet at some point it is open to us to decide that we can live well enough with and on a ragged edge, that we need not always try to get rid of it. We can make such a decision in general about pushing back the frontiers of aging (settling, say, for our present average life span), or about particular diseases and harmful conditions (deciding, say, to stop research on how to save babies weighing less than 500 grams at birth). Or we can decide (as I will argue in Chapter 4) that we already have a sufficiently good level of healthcare and reduce our general efforts at still greater improvement. Why stop here and now? Because we have already come a long way and because the economic and social costs of continuing to push on have become intolerably high.

We should be prepared to make such decisions, knowing perfectly well that some lives will be lost at that ragged edge we decide to accept and not to overcome. We can accept it, not because we lack sympathy for those on it, but because we know that, once a ragged edge is defeated, we will then simply move on to still another ragged edge, with new victims— and there will always be new victims. It is a struggle we cannot win, but can harm ourselves trying to win. We can, instead, turn to a different goal. We can ask not how to continually push back all frontiers, smooth out all ragged edges, but how to make life tolerable on the ragged edges; for we will all one day be on such an edge, sooner or later. We can ask how best to live on such frontiers, how best to care for each other there. We cannot get rid of the ragged edge of individual cure, but we might come to some understanding about how to live with it, to make it tolerable, if never fully acceptable.

## THE NEED FOR CARE: CHANGING OUR WAY OF LIFE

I have made a strong case against the goal of meeting individual curative need as the highest aim of the healthcare system. I have tried to show it is neither feasible nor even meaningful. It is, however, an objection to the *concept* of "individual need," not to the moral aspiration to respect individuals. I do not want in any sense to imply that we should abandon the individual. That is not economically necessary, morally acceptable, or politically plausible. But the impossibility of meeting individual curative needs means that we will have to significantly alter our understanding and expectations about how the individual can best be respected, served, and helped by the healthcare system. If our present understanding of individual need is set in a way of life that is dedicated to self-determination and self-definition, and restless with any limits to the frontiers of what the self wants in the name of health and longevity, then it is ultimately that way of life that must be questioned and changed. Our medical and health values are of a piece with many of our other cultural and political values—the centrality of the individual, the use of the language of rights to pursue our private welfare, the belief that limits on the possibilities of human nature need not be accepted—and thus they must be dealt with together.

Let me take here the first steps in sketching an alternative direction. Implicit in my analysis so far has been a focus on the need for *cure*. We look to contemporary medicine to make us better, to save us from death, and to cure our diseases and disabilities—what I have called curative medicine. It is that sense of meeting individual need that I have tried to expose for what it is: a recipe for endlessly increased expenditures and perpetually needy, dissatisfied people.

There is an alternative. We could make the societal priority the meeting of our need for *care* rather than for cure. While the need for caring can be extensive, costly, and burdensome, it does not have about it the inherently open-ended features that mark the need for cure. If all of the needs of the body for cure cannot be met, as they can never be, the emotional and social needs of the person whose body is sick can usually be met to some minimally adequate extent. That effort does not require endless technological innovation, or constant breakthroughs on the frontiers of research. It requires that adequate provision be made to relieve pain, to provide institutional and home care when family resources fail, and to provide counseling and support in the face of suffering. What caring requires, for the most part, is concern and sympathy, time and personal attention. There will still be a ragged edge—some people will be beyond effective caring, and some forms of the relief of suffering may require technological advancement—but of much smaller, potentially manageable magnitude.

The provision of caring will become all the more important in an era increasingly dominated by chronic illness, where patients do not at once die, or necessarily show progressive decline, but where their disease becomes a permanent part of their life.[32] For those in the worst condition, institutional care will be needed, or home care for those less worse off. They must be helped to live with their disease and the institutions of society must be shaped in ways that give support to these individuals in their illness. For the elderly, this kind of support will be vital. We will not be able to pursue with the elderly the cure of every condition to which the body in its aging is subject, or to provide an infinite amount of life-extending care (which is, by definition, the amount needed to meet the body needs of the elderly). What we can do, however, is to provide decent nursing-home care, home care, and a wide range of drugs and devices which, while they will not extend life, will make life much more tolerable.

The first priority of clinical medicine and the healthcare system, therefore, should be to ensure that everyone has an adequate level of caring. For the bodily ill, this will mean the relief of pain and good nursing care. For the psychologically ill, this will mean counseling, palliative care and, when necessary, decent institutional care. For those who are disabled, handicapped, or retarded, it will mean assistance with the activities of daily living, help in adapting to their environment, and good institutional care if neither they nor their families are able to manage their care. The provision of a minimal baseline of caring, and just what it might require, will need discussion and debate—and that debate will require a recognition of limits on care. I will develop the place of caring further in Chapter 5, when I consider the establishment of societal priorities for healthcare. First, however, it is necessary to look more closely at the ideal of efficiency.

# CHAPTER 3

# HOPES, VAIN HOPES: THE PURSUIT OF EFFICIENCY

What is there about those whose lives are constant failures, whose every effort at change comes to nothing? At first we are tempted to go along with their explanations. They made a mistake in their investment. They loved the wrong person. They should have taken the other job. Then we begin to wonder. Why do they keep losing their money, falling damagingly in love again and again, choosing once more a dead-end job? They resist having this pattern pointed out to them. We are, they say, making too much of coincidence. But are we? Is the pattern of misfortune just chance?

The American healthcare system presents such a case. For nearly two decades it has tried to provide more efficient care. Yet it has failed to do either and continues to fail. Is it just an accident or coincidence? No. It is of the very nature of our present system to maldistribute care and to drive up costs. It is not actually a system at all, but a collection of programs and disparate institutions, neither coherently conceived nor coherently operated. Efforts to achieve any significant efficiency reforms by the most commonly employed—and commonly venerated—methods are *inevitably* bound to fail. Those methods, a combination of incentives and disincentives, carrots and sticks, make use of false perceptions and faulty premises. They want to manipulate into good behavior a fundamentally deranged system, one whose problems mount with each passing year.

To call our system "deranged" may seem harsh.[1] It is, after all, one that sought in the years following World War II to create a superb plan of biomedical research, and soon after began the quest for the world's highest-quality medical care. When it became clear, moreover, that many people could not afford the new medical advances and the growing cost of healthcare, strong efforts were made to bring equity into the system. The Medicare program for the elderly, and the Medicaid plan for the poor, both passed by Congress in 1965, were important steps toward a more just system and eventually, many hoped, toward a full national health insurance scheme.[2] When it became evident, finally, by the early 1970s that healthcare costs were increasing at a disturbing pace, efforts were undertaken to control costs and promote greater efficiency.

Out of the drive for the three goals of quality, equity, and efficiency grew a powerful faith, one that sustains the system to this day. It is the belief that the needs of each and every individual can be met with high-quality healthcare if that care can be organized and delivered in an efficient way—and that can be done without a change of fundamental values. This conviction has assumed that the key to meeting individual need is greater biomedical knowledge and the steady advance of technological medicine. No less powerful is the certainty that advances in technology will eventually reduce costs, and that medical progress and medical efficiency are perfectly compatible values. This set of convictions rests on a still deeper belief that in health affairs people should get what they want and think they need; and what they want is acceptable because there can be no common social standard by which to judge health wants and demands. We cannot as a society tell people how long they ought to want to live, it is widely held, or with what quality of life they should be prepared to live. There is no substantive view of the human good to guide us, other than meeting whatever preferences individuals express and we can collectively afford. With sufficient efficiency, it nicely happens, we can in any event collectively afford whatever it is we now want and will come to want in the future.

Most of those beliefs and convictions are false. We cannot pursue a limitless idea of quality and hope to do so efficiently. We cannot achieve both maximum quality and full equity. If we are to have both equity and efficiency, then we must change our notions of quality. If we are to have both efficiency and quality, we must change our ideas about equity. Most of all, we must come to understand that, if we are to achieve both efficiency and equity, we must give up, or significantly modify, some long-standing values, notably that of individual choice to meet individual needs. Neither efficiency nor equity can be achieved by that route. Our present system rests upon an incoherent set of values and is embedded in a way of life guaranteeing its failure.

## THE QUEST FOR THE BEST

In the years immediately following World War II, no nation on earth came to believe so hopefully and steadfastly in the value and necessity of good health as the United States. At least through the late 1960s, Congress was willing to allocate to research and healthcare whatever it seemed to take to have "the best" system in the world. And it appeared to work. For some years now, there has been widespread national self-congratulation that the United States has the best medicine in the world.

On what does that claim appear to rest? In the National Institutes of Health (NIH) the United States has the preeminent biomedical research organization, and not only because of the research carried out internally by the NIH, but also because its system of grant support for external research is unmatched. With an annual investment of over $7 billion a year, it does more for biomedical research both in the United States and throughout the world than any similar organization. The consequences of that strong research base can be seen in the advanced state of American medical technology. It has provided leadership in organ transplantation, pharmaceuticals, intensive care for patients, and the quality of its medical researchers. American medical schools are among the best, and the teaching hospitals affiliated with those schools are well known for the quality of their training; for decades they have drawn physicians and researchers from all over the world to work in them. Those hospitals are unparalleled for the quality of their care and for their employment of the most advanced technology.

Closely examined, the boast that the American system is "the best" mainly comes down to its development and deployment of high-technology medicine.[3] The claim is that the measure of the best care is the availability of the most advanced technological methods of diagnosis, cure, and rehabilitation. In that respect, one can readily point to the fruit of decades of research, the large amount of money invested in past years for the improvement of sophisticated technologies, and their availability in the most advanced institutions. The measure, then, is not the rounded capacities and strengths of the system, but the strengths of its strength—that of the availability of technological devices that most save life and provide dramatic cures.

If the American system is thought to be the best in the world, why can it be said that the United States has a crisis in healthcare? The most palpable reason is the discrepancy between the best being available for some, in some places, and being dismally poor or unavailable for many millions in other places (often in the next block). At the same time as that discrepancy exists, and grows, the cost of healthcare is rising at a rapid and unacceptable rate. The combination of erratic care and coverage, together with uncontrolled costs, puts the claim that the United States has "the best" system in a different light. As Uwe E. Reinhardt has written, "At its best, the American health system is unmatched anywhere in the world. At its worst, no other industrialized nation would ever want to match it."[4] The problems of the system can roughly be divided into two categories: those bearing on the large gaps in health insurance now being experienced, and those bearing on the cost of medical treatment.

Some 35 million to 40 million Americans lack health insurance, and many millions beyond that have inadequate insurance. In the late 1970s, the number of uninsured Americans reached a low of 13 percent, but since that time it has risen close to 18 percent, and that trend continues (with children making up 32 percent of the uninsured).[5] A basic reason for the large number of uninsured is the lack of any organized national system of health insurance and the failure of many American businesses to offer their employees health coverage. That situation has been exacerbated by a variety of discouraging developments in recent years. Most notably, a number of states have tightened their eligibility criteria for Medicaid; only 40 percent of those with incomes below the federal poverty line are now covered by Medicaid (compared with 63 percent in 1975).[6] The recession of the early 1980s created a larger pool of people living and remaining below the poverty line, estimated to have increased by some 37 percent, or 10 million people. The fact that many of the post-recession jobs have been primarily in the service sector, together with the continuing and sharp annual rise in insurance premiums, has meant that many working people are unable to afford insurance. Between an absence of insurance and the difficulty of qualifying for Medicaid, they are desperately at risk from illnesses that may both ruin their bodies and devastate their finances.

Beyond those who are simply uninsured or ineligible for Medicaid, there are many millions of middle-class Americans whose insurance provides inadequate protection, particularly against catastrophic illness. That kind of illness can well devour a family's resources, and does so for thousands each year. For specific at-risk groups of the population, minorities and the poor, the shortcomings of the system are all the more evident. The necessity that, under Medicaid regulations, families impoverish themselves before qualifying for long-term nursing-home care is a well-publicized failing of the healthcare system for the elderly, but also for younger people as well. For those elderly living alone, seven out of ten are at risk of being impoverished by long-term care within thirteen weeks of admission to a nursing home.[7] Even for families fortunate enough to be able to afford the average of $20,000 to $30,000 a year for nursing-home care, the rapid depletion of resources accumulated over a lifetime or the demands that can sometimes be made upon children with families of their own are a source of stress, sadness, and sometimes outright tragedy. Although a solid program for long-term care has been a primary goal of a number of advocacy groups among the elderly, particularly the American Association of Retired Persons, there is a great deal of wariness in Congress about its potential costs, estimated between $20 billion and $40 billion a year.[8] (See Table 6, p. 273.) The same is true of the need for better home care to relieve families of the psychological and physical burdens of care for the elderly, and sometimes the incidental financial burdens as well.

The general pressures to control costs add to a widespread sense of malaise throughout the system. In 1975–1980 the percentage of gross national product devoted to healthcare rose by 0.8 percentage point, from 8.4 to 9.2 percent. But this was comparatively slight compared with the changes that were in the offing—1.5 percent increase over the next five years, 9.2 percent in 1980 to 10.7 percent in 1985. By 1987, some 11.1 percent of the GNP was devoted to healthcare. Medicare payments for hospital care went from $25.9 billion to $50.9 billion between 1980 and 1987, a 100 percent increase; and Medicare costs for physicians increased by 179 percent during the same period.[9] By comparison, in 1985 the 10.7 percent of the American GNP devoted to healthcare was higher than the 9.4 percent of Sweden, the 8.4 percent of Canada, the 8.2 percent of West Germany, and the 6.1 percent of Great Britain. The United States spends 2.8 times as much per capita on healthcare as Great Britain (with essentially identical health outcomes though with better amenities and shorter waiting times in the United States), 1.7 times as much as the French, 1.5 times as much as the Swedes, and 1.4 times as much as Canada. In 1986, when the general rate of inflation had dropped to 1.1 percent, healthcare costs rose by 7.7 percent and they have remained in that range since then.[10]

At the same time as these general costs were out of control, proof against all efforts to hold them down, a closer look at the system revealed some equally disturbing figures. With corporations, for example, it was found that some 15 percent of employees account for 90 percent of healthcare costs, with a particularly sharp increase in the number of medical claims in the $50,000–$100,000 range.[11] This has been brought about by the increased coverage of organ and bone-marrow transplantation, neonatal care, mental health care, and the proliferation of such procedures as coronary bypass surgery. For corporations, claims in 1986 for procedures costing over $100,000 increased by 33 percent, signaling a decisive trend in the direction of ever more expensive high-technology procedures. The "vertical gap" (noted in Chapter 2) becomes all the more pronounced.

## THE FAILURE OF COST CONTAINMENT

A large number of initiatives, dating well back to the advent of Medicare and Medicaid in the mid-1960s, have tried to deal with the dual problem of the uninsured and the containment of costs.[12] With minor qualifications, they can all be judged as failures. At no point have the problems been unnoticed, and at no point has there been an absence of proposals to deal with both of them. Up through the mid-1970s there was a push for national health insurance, but it faded in the face of increasing healthcare costs. By the late 1970s cost containment became the central focus. Though cost containment efforts had first begun with the Nixon administration in 1970, it was not until the end of that decade that the intensity of concern reached a high pitch. One scheme after another was introduced to hold down costs.[13]

Most of the reforms of the 1970s and 1980s have been major disappointments. Efforts to contain costs have failed to accomplish their ultimate goal of significantly curbing excessive increases, and not because of failure to admit the existence of a problem. Healthcare costs have continued to increase at a pace approximately double that of general inflation, 7–9 percent versus 4–5 percent, and the situation has become worse in the past few years, not better.[14] That waste, excessive and unnecessary diagnostic procedures, and useless or only marginally beneficial treatments are widespread is acknowledged. No less admitted is a profound incapacity so far to diminish them. In the face of this dismal record it is easy to simply say that there has not been a political seriousness or a genuine regulatory zeal to manage costs—that it has "not really been tried." There is surely some truth in that perception, but a much more likely possibility is that all of the solutions tried so far have had failure built into them, and that it is inevitable that like techniques in the future will continue to fail without some far-reaching changes in underlying values. There will surely be some successes, but it seems unlikely they will be sufficient to make a decisive difference. Our problem is not that we lack clever ideas to increase health insurance coverage, or to control costs, but that there is a failure at a more profound level to understand the momentum of our system, and particularly the way a number of characteristic American values increase costs and inhibit controls.

The collapse of the cost-containment movement provides a superb window into the internal inconsistencies, contradictions, and profound confusions of the system as a whole. To be sure, without that movement, the situation might have been worse. But that is small consolation, more helpful to the search for a silver lining than to effective cost containment.[15] Whether the focus is on such strategies as prepaid programs, competition, outpatient care, corporate insurance rates, or the general inflationary costs of care, the results have been consistently poor regardless of the nature of the strategy.

The three principal means of cost containment have been the encouragement of competition, the promotion of health maintenance organizations (HMOs), and the control of hospital reimbursements under Medicare. Competition between and among healthcare providers, for instance—pressed by the Reagan administration in its early years—has been a notable failure.[16] While having a theoretical capacity to lower costs, competition can actually increase the desire of people for more care by loudly calling attention to their health risks and needs, and by an expansion or intensification of the range of services promoted once they seek it. It serves, that is, to stimulate, not dampen, medical and health expectations. That should hardly have come as a shock. The competitive market system that we know as capitalism in the United States has been supported precisely because it is thought to foster growth, prosperity, and income. The belief that those same forces in the case of the healthcare system could be used to reduce prosperity, to bring down costs, and to keep budgets within control was a triumph of hope over logic. That dynamic, interacting with the way the system is internally organized, all but guarantees an increase in cost, and generated from the inside, not just the outside.

The hopes vested in the HMO movement show a similar lack of insight into the ways things work. It was assumed that HMOs would provide self-contained care systems, where the costs could well be managed by internal staff and technological discipline. As it happens, however, the same attitudes that exist in the larger society are readily brought into the HMO system: expensive physician and patient choices, high technological expectations, and bureaucratic inefficiencies. In order to gain and keep patients, moreover, HMOs are very often forced to compete with each other by offering superior service, a practice that increases costs. The many HMOs in financial difficulty, the general slowing of the growth of HMOs, the dissatisfaction with the way many are managed, and the quality of care they provide have all served to dampen the early enthusiasm for their cost-containing potential.[17]

The failure of the system of diagnosis-related groups (DRGs) under the Medicare program, expected to hold down hospital costs, is similarly instructive. While that system has been effective in reducing the number of hospital days, shortening the stay of patients in hospitals, it has not succeeded in bringing down costs in general.[18] The money saved in hospital care has more than been spent in an increased use of critical-care nursing facilities, for those now discharged earlier from hospitals than had been typical, and in the increased use of outpatient facilities and services. The DRG system has so far mainly shifted the costs from one sector to another, with no apparent net gain in savings.

I do not want to deny the possibility of finding some *relatively* effective approaches to cost containment, or the need to keep trying. Recent reports suggest the DRG system may be having an effect on costs. The technique of utilization review (screening before hospital admission, for instance) is a promising method, and others will doubtless be found. More generally, a new wave of hope is being invested in "managed care" and "managed competition," led by Stanford economist Alain Enthoven. "The essence of *managed competition*," he writes, "is the use of available tools to structure cost-conscious consumer choice in the pursuit of equity and efficiency in healthcare financing and delivery."[19] There is no reason, however, to think that this new variant on an old idea will be sufficient to the magnitude of the task at hand, much less to the task to be faced in the future as the number of elderly grows. Managed care programs are not likely as now conceived to cope with the full scope of the economic problem, a problem generated in great part by a system badly ridden with internal contradictions.[20] It is hard to fault the judgment of the distinguished economist Eli Ginzberg in his conclusion, "Until we approach the upper limit of acceptable health care expenditures . . . cost containment is likely to remain the elusive hare that the hounds pursue but never overtake"; or to take issue with Dr. William B. Schwartz in his even starker conclusion that cost containment, at its best, can provide only temporary relief to cost increase.[21]

The most basic contradiction is that at the same time that we desire to control costs, we want also to improve the quality and extent of, and access to, healthcare. At the same time that we are trying to reduce the cost of entitlement programs, such as Medicare, we are bringing organ transplantation and other forms of high-technology care under those programs. At the same time that we talk of death with dignity, we increase the budgets to cure all known causes of death. At the same time that we talk about the need for justice and equal access, we work to preserve and extend individual choice and opportunity. At the same time that we try to contain costs, and avoid rationing, we continue to affirm those values that drive up costs.

## A TRIPLE DYNAMIC: AGE, TECHNOLOGY, DEMAND

I believe it is an error to see in those contradictions nothing more than irrationality, narrow self-interest, and shortsightedness. Doubtless they are present, and in good measure, but then they are present in most human affairs. The problem here is more profound. It is a striking instance of what happens when we as a people pursue high goals (improving health, delaying death) and live out otherwise high values in pursuing them (personal freedom and self-determination), but fail to understand that they have unleashed a combination of biological and social forces with incalculable consequences. Those forces, it turns out, are neither easily understandable nor, once unleashed, readily controllable; and that invites illusions, evasions, and contradictions. We cannot live with or afford our ideals, but neither can we readily give them up or modify them.

There are three biological and social factors of central consequence that together constitute a potent force. One of them is the reality of an aging population in general and a rapidly increasing proportion of elderly in particular. (See table 7, p. 274.) The approximately 30 million people over the age of sixty-five, some 12 percent of the population, are projected to double within the next thirty years, to make up close to 20 percent of the population. The fastest-growing age group is those over the age of eighty-five, and their number could well triple over the same period. With that increase will come a growing demand for improved healthcare, bound to put severe stress on the health-care system. The second reality, more social than biological, is the unrelenting drive for improved medical technology. The working assumption of modern medicine is that biological research creates knowledge of a kind that, through technological application, can be translated into clinical practice, and that, whatever the present state of understanding and technology, it can be improved, made ever better. The third reality, political and cultural, is that of a powerful, unremitting public demand for better health and a longer life. This public demand is fueled by a natural desire for good health, by the earlier success of medicine in providing it, by the promise of new knowledge and technology in improving it, and by the belief that the more choices people have about their health and their lives the better off they will be.

The power of this triple force—age, technology, demand— is greatly magnified by the pervasive beliefs in our culture that it is good to live a long, even longer life; that it is good to use the mind and the economy in devising ways to cure disease and control death; and that it is good to give people choice about the fate of their health and their bodies. It is a dynamic, in short, that rests upon high and long-revered values. For just that reason any serious effort at rethinking and reforming the healthcare system must begin with an examination of those values. Most reform efforts, and particularly the cost-containment movement, have wanted to change the mechanics of the system while preserving its fundamental values. The problem has been taken to be one of means, not ends. But just that emphasis is why reform efforts have failed, and will continue to fail. Serious efforts at efficiency will require a ready willingness to change, modify, and compromise those values. One need only look at the system with a sharp eye to see that.

The healthcare industry in the United States, for example, is highly profitable, feeding effectively upon public desire and demand, and in turn helping to stimulate that desire and demand. The aggregate costs of technology increase in great part because they are commercially designed to increase: Improved products are constantly brought on the market, wider patient populations are sought for the available technologies, and older technologies are updated so that they will not be displaced by newer ones (and thus to be supplemented, not evicted, by newer technologies). Yet it is a profound mistake to blame industry alone for this state of affairs. It is giving the public what it demands, and what it demands is better health, a process that feeds upon itself. The growth of an aging population, for instance, has meant an increase in chronic illness (even if it may be leveling off with the very old).[22] (See Table 4, p. 271.) The larger the number of people saved by acute, high-technology medicine, the larger the number of those who are going to bear some degree of disability and require ongoing acute care and rehabilitation. That process in turn stimulates the need for even more technology, to improve the lives now extended.

Better health, it happens, raises expectations for still better health, and that in turn requires improved technology. The healthcare industry generates through its success its own market. It is profitable not simply because people are willing to pay for it, but also because it allows them to have an increasingly long life in which to desire more of it. Technological medicine is a dream in this setting, promising to give everyone what they want and helping to tell them just what it is they should want. It is a rich, self-fertilizing world, and not one congenial to serious cost containment.

The expanding domain of medicine is no less important a force in working against cost containment. There has been an increase in recent years in the demand for better mental health and a consequent expansion of services and benefits, and a no less powerful drive to bring substance addiction and abuse within the medical realm. This general expansion of the scope of healthcare—well beyond traditional medical boundaries into areas that would once have been handled by the criminal law or the social welfare system—is as unlimited in its expansionary possibilities as the management of physical and psychological ills. Here, before our eyes, we can see what it means to live out the WHO definition of health, now well buried but fully alive in our culture.

# THE DESIRE FOR "QUALITY"

To the expanded scope of medicine has been added a fresh focus on the preservation and improvement of "quality" in the provision of healthcare. A commonly expressed goal is that of high-quality healthcare at reasonable and affordable costs. Yet "quality" as ordinarily used is an inherently expansive and elastic concept, one incapable of being fully distinguished from the values and interests of those making judgments about it. A simple, but plausible, definition of "high-quality" care is that "the highest quality medical care is that care that best achieves legitimate medical and non-medical goals."[23] That definition well shows, however, how subject "quality" will be to contending goals. Just what is "best" and what is "legitimate"? Patients, medical practitioners, and corporate or institutional purchasers of care are all likely to have different definitions, as befits their different perspectives.[24] That a good bit of renewed concern for "quality" among practitioners is a response to the perceived threat of cost containment seems likely. Nonetheless, efficacy of treatment, its appropriateness for a particular condition, and its provision under conditions of caring for, and sensitivity to, patients are some core, relatively disinterested criteria for "quality."[25]

The problem is to embody such values in the provision of healthcare in a way that makes them help, not directly hinder, the containment of costs. That means understanding quality in a way that does not entail constant improvement of outcomes and the raising of standards; that is, avoiding inherently expansionary notions of "quality." At present, however, the quest for "quality" most often serves as an obstacle, an expression of the triumph of aspiration, desire, profit, and ambition over control and restraint. The dismay that greets any evidence of a decline in quality as a result of efforts at efficiency and cost containment is revelatory.[26] It shows the persistence of the myth that costs can be controlled with no serious pain or sacrifice. Our entire way of life economically and politically—as summed up nicely by the desire for ever-improving "quality"—is based on the growth and expansion, not the contraction, of demand and expenditure.

Some profound value commitments at the very heart of our political and moral system abet these expansionist tendencies. The long-standing, and traditional, tension between freedom and justice works powerfully here as well as in other areas of American life.[27] But the weight of the tension is usually resolved in the direction of freedom, and that dominant commitment means that people are allowed, indeed encouraged, to expand their horizons, to increase their expectations, and to define in any way that is personally congenial to them what it means to have a need. If they are aggrieved when services are denied them, or corners cut on quality, the courts are readily available to them, and litigation to assert individual rights against societal demands is common.

Choice is, in the end, king. As the authors of *Critical Condition* put it—by way of commending a supposed strength of our system—"consumers have more choices about their care than ever before."[28] But it is precisely that kind of a benefit of the system that is itself at the root of our problem. Nothing is more potent in driving up costs than the quest for unlimited improvement in quality combined with an unlimited desire to maximize choice, and then setting this combination in a system that is not a system. While the values of justice and freedom are promoted and touted, the fact of the matter is that in any strong showdown between the two forces, it is typically freedom—more and more individual choice—that is the winner. In the case of the health-care system this has meant an exultation of the freedom of providers to provide quality care as they define such care, and for consumers to seek the best possible care, and where and how they choose to define it as well.[29] The quest for quality, defined ordinarily as improved technology, works very closely with a quest for individual freedom of choice. And it works directly against cost containment.

The depth of the problem here is evident from public-opinion surveys. They show, in general, that the public rates good health close to the top of personal aspirations and that it wants improved public and private programs of healthcare.

Quality is a major public concern. The surveys also show, however, that the public is unwilling to consider any significant increase in taxes to pay for the improvement and quality desired. This profound ambivalence, even contradiction, indicates that we are at a painful psychological and ethical impasse, one whose force is played out as a powerful undercurrent in cost-containment efforts. Two studies of public opinion—one by Louis Harris and Associates for the Loran Commission, and the other by the Public Agenda Foundation—help reveal why there is so much confusion.

In the 1987 Harris survey, some 74 percent of the general public said they were willing to see more spent on healthcare, and an impressive 91 percent said that "everybody should have the right to get the best possible healthcare—as good as the treatment a millionaire gets."[30] Not only does the public want splendid healthcare for all, by a significant majority (66 to 31 percent) it also holds that "it's not fair that some people can afford to buy more and better health insurance than others."[31] An even higher proportion (71 to 26 percent) believe that "health insurance should pay for any treatments that will save lives even if it costs one million dollars to save a life."[32]

Yet those generous sentiments are a bit too good to be the whole truth. A large majority recognize (by an 80 to 17 percent margin) that even if we radically increased what is now spent on healthcare, we could still not provide all the services people would like to have. They also recognize (by a 76 to 22 percent margin) that the constant appearance of new and very expensive ways of treating the sick will soon force harsh choices. The public, in brief, knows that we are not likely to achieve an ideal of universal access to all desired healthcare. People also know that the system as a whole requires change. Their idealism is tempered by realism; some limitations are understood to be necessary and acceptable. The public, moreover, also believes that we do not receive a good value for the money we now spend on healthcare, and thinks we could have a more efficient system.

The Harris survey ends on a positive note, stressing the power of public discussion to change attitudes and, especially, to make the public more realistic about what can be accomplished. "A public debate," the survey concludes, "would be likely to increase . . . the number of people who feel that it is not only inevitable, but reasonable, that health plans limit their coverage in order to stay within finite resources."[33] That is an optimistic conclusion, grounded in changes noted in the survey respondents themselves as a result of participation in the study.

The findings of the Public Agenda Foundation at first seem to parallel those of the Harris survey.[34] Asking a somewhat narrower set of questions—would the public favor a government program to cover catastrophic illness, even if the estimated cost ran to $10 billion a year?—the study found a strong majority in approval. There was widespread recognition that catastrophic illness could bankrupt a family, and that it was a danger for all families and not just poor ones. There was a corresponding belief that it is the duty of government, not families, to bear the cost of such illness. So far so good.

But the Public Agenda study pushed one step further, and the mood rapidly changed. It pressed its respondents—a sociologically solid population sample—to see if they would be willing to pay the taxes necessary to support the catastrophic illness program. The answer was no: "Only about 1 in 10 of the respondents said they would agree to a tax increase of roughly $125/year—the proposal's estimated cost for the average taxpayer—for this purpose."[35] This is a sobering outcome, dampening the hope for public reasonableness that was present in the Harris survey. Worse still, the findings of the Public Agenda Foundation came after extended discussion and "time to ponder the problem"; the responses were not casual or unconsidered. Their study concludes, "As concerned as they were about their vulnerability to the high cost of catastrophic illness and long-term care . . . most of the participants . . . remained unwilling either to lower their own expectations about what the government should provide, or to pay what is necessary for even a modest level of government-provided coverage. . . . While there is strong support for more government involvement in this area, there is no corresponding inclination to pay for it."[36]

This ought to be a chilling piece of information for those who have long cherished the belief that the public is willing to pay more for good healthcare. It is also suggestive in helping us think about the failures of cost containment. It indicates at the least that the correlation between high public expectations about healthcare and the failure of cost containment efforts is not coincidence. While the Harris survey notes some tempering realism about the possibility of unlimited healthcare, that realism does not yet seem strong enough to overcome the wishful thinking about health insurance that emerged from the deeper probing of the Public Agenda study. If the public shows little willingness to curb its desires for more and better healthcare, how can we reasonably expect that serious, demanding cost containment efforts will be sustained? There is at work here a profound power of denial and a baffling willingness to live with unresolved contradiction, perhaps a legacy of the high expectations stimulated by available health insurance in the 1960s and 1970s when difficult choices were not necessary. As a perceptive 1984 article noted, "The public shows only limited interest in cost–containment proposals that are seen as requiring them to change substantially the way in which they receive . . . care."[37]

## ILLUSIONS OF NECESSITY— INTERNATIONAL LESSONS

The power of denial runs deeply here, often among professionals no less than among the public. The most important kind of denial is that which believes that the desired combination of efficiency, effective cost containment, and high-quality care can be had without a significant sacrifice of fundamental values, notably those of steady medical progress, improved health, and expanded choice. This belief has sustained itself of late with two sources of nourishment. The first is the example of other developed nations, which have provided good healthcare to their citizens at a much lower cost per capita and with a much lower share of their GNP devoted to healthcare. The Canadian experience has in particular been invoked as a salubrious instance of what can be done. If they can do it, the argument goes, so can we.

Canadian health economist Robert G. Evans has helped to bring the experience of other countries into sharp focus, and particularly the Canadian situation. There are, he has argued, "illusions of necessity" about the forces of an aging society and technological developments.[38] They need not necessarily lead to higher costs, as if driven by some intrinsic necessity. Everything depends upon the response to them, and that is under human control. It is, for instance, the intensification of services to the elderly that has increased costs so sharply, not the number of elderly as such. As for the supposed driving force of technological development, Evans points out that while it has increased costs in the United States, it has not done so correspondingly in Canada. The difference lies in the incentives within the American system for the proliferation of more intensive technological interventions as well as a reimbursement bias toward those new technologies that increase costs.

Evans is making a profound and important point. It is true that no "necessity" lies behind the costs attributed to aging and technology; it is human beings, through their choices and systems, that cause things to happen. Yet that is not quite the whole truth either. Demographic trends and technological developments are set within the values of a culture, chosen by that culture, and it is those values that will determine the response to them. In the American setting, the combination of age and technology has led to a demand for an intensification of services that has driven up the costs. We demand that aging be fought against. There is, so to speak, a necessity about the application of some profound American values to the fact of an aging society and technological developments. It is not the age and technology that create the necessity, but the way our national values shape the response to them. The Canadian values are different, but that makes all the difference, and no one has shown how the deeply seated Canadian values (a willingness to accept government controls and a greater coolness toward technological progress) can be transferred across the border to displace the no less deeply rooted American values (resistance to regulation and love of technology).[39]

Yet there may be an even more important reality now emerging. Canada and other European countries have managed to control the costs of healthcare in a way that Americans can only envy, and they have done so in a way that has maintained a level of health as good as that in the United States. But their success may also be running out. As the editors of a 1984 study of healthcare in the Western industrialized nations observed, "The notion that the welfare state can provide an abundance of health services for all its citizens is an illusion. In the future, social policy is likely to veer from idealism to realism, from opportunity to constraint."[40] That prediction has taken some years to be borne out, but with proposals to reform the British National Health Service, and discussion about rationing in Sweden and elsewhere, it may now be happening. The cloud on the horizon is from the same storm that has afflicted the United States, that of "intensity of services," the application of more technology and service to individual patients. As George J. Schieber and Jean-Pierre Poulier have noted, "Even countries that appear to have mastered the problem of excessive health care inflation face significant increases in per capita utilization/intensity of services."[41] There has also been a steadily growing concern about the impact of an aging population and the increasingly large proportion of elderly, a point that Evans himself has noted in commenting on the future of the Canadian system.[42] More generally, public knowledge of and demand for technological improvements have grown in other countries, as has the demand for greater patient choice. In comparison with Americans, Europeans have characteristically been less demanding and fractious as patients, more willing to accept limits to care, less addicted to the latest technology.

All that seems now in the process of changing, and there is good reason to believe that many values thought idiosyncratic to the United States are spreading. The American "illusions of necessity" may become everyone's illusions. The attraction of technological progress as a cultural ideal, for a long time uniquely powerful in the United States because of its ready liaison with the individualism of American culture, is now a potent international force, and so also with it increased demand for individual choice. While it may long have been the case that the American problem with its healthcare system was unique among developed, affluent countries, the problems of other developed countries show signs of becoming more like ours, not the other way around.

## ILLUSIONS OF SALVATION— ASSESSING TECHNOLOGY

The second way denial has been nourished is through the conviction that, since a wasteful use of technology is at the heart of our inefficient medicine, tough programs of technology assessment and clinical efficacy can correct that error. Yet while the role of medical technology in the rising cost of healthcare has long been known, it is hard to think of any area of healthcare at once so full of hopeful proposals and in fact so highly resistant to change and control. Over the past two decades the estimates of the relative inflationary role of technology have ranged from 20 to 40 percent, with "little-ticket" items (lab tests, ECGs, etc.) being most responsible for increases in the 1960s and early 1970s and "big-ticket" items (CAT scans, for example) for increases in the 1980s.[43] It is nonetheless said that it is both desirable and possible to reduce the cost of technology. The simple fact of the matter, however, is that while the cost of discrete technologies can be reduced—either the costs for individual users or the costs per unit of the technology, or both—the history of the introduction and spread of medical technologies in this country has been to drive up *aggregate* costs.

Just as it is by no means the case that an old technology is invariably dropped when a new one appears, it is also typically the case that, as the price per unit of the use of technology drops, the population of potential users of the technology increases.

That has been the story of the VCR, the microwave oven, and the personal computer, to take some obvious examples in our personal lives, and the phenomenon is equally pervasive in health-care. A desire to expand the overall market for a medical technology is a powerful incentive to reduce unit costs. Few institutions can afford devices that cost $1 million, and the market for them will remain small. If the cost of the same device can be brought down to $50,000 then every institution can have one, and more than one. It should hardly astonish us then that there is simply no evidence, in this or any other society, that a widespread and diligent use of technology brings down costs in general, even if it brings some discrete and isolated savings here and there. It is part of the nature of our system, on the contrary, to look to technological advances as the main way of increasing our prosperity and gross national product. An investment in research and development is taken to be a key ingredient of sustained economic growth, which is in the end nothing more than more income to buy more goods. As Robert G. Evans has noted, "Technological innovations that *really* reduce costs, simultaneously and by definition reduce sales and income as well."[44]

There have been responses to these general objections. The first is that it is not technology that is the culprit but "the degree to which the deployment of new medical technology reflects legitimate consumer demand for higher quality care."[45] But that is precisely the problem—the desire for care of ever higher quality, which makes real control of costs all but impossible, and the belief that the desire is "legitimate," which undercuts any solid reason to resist the technology. What is by critics called "medical excess" is, by defenders, translated into an acceptable expression of "widespread patient and professional demand for greater technological research and sophistication."[46] Which is exactly why we have a problem.

Another response to criticisms of the cost of medical technologies is that not only does a concentration on the aggregate costs of technology overlook the contribution of individual technologies to cost reduction, but a more long-term view is needed.

Such a view would suggest, for example, that "for heart disease and cancer, new tests and treatments may be capable of lowering the indirect cost of disease more than they increase direct outlays. Thus the 'total cost pie' would shrink, even as the intensity of the medical care slice grew relatively larger. . . . From this perspective, technology becomes a tool to produce long-term social value, rather than an inflationary entity to be controlled. The historical focus . . . on technology as additive to direct costs of care did not take this concept into account."[47] But "this concept" is, at bottom, wholly speculative in its potentiality to lower the system costs and little more than a plea to look favorably upon technology as a source of "social value." Perhaps so, but not an inexpensive source.

Yet if general assurances that technological developments will one day or another serve to restrain costs ring increasingly hollow, more substantial hopes have been invested in technology assessment. Though hardly new, technology assessment has now become the method of choice for managing the costs of technological medicine. Its premise is simple and seemingly commonsensical. If we can only discover what works well— which diagnostic procedures and tests, which operations and treatments are efficacious and cost effective—we can then eliminate useless or excessively costly, minimally effective technologies. Or, as the Office of Technology Assessment of the U.S. Congress more formally defined it, "Medical technology assessment is, in a narrow sense, the evaluation or testing of a medical technology for safety and efficacy. In a broader sense, it is a process of policy research that examines the short- and long-term consequences of individual medical technologies."[48] It is hard to argue with such a laudable goal, and it is surely valuable to determine which tests and procedures are effective and what the relative harms and benefits, and implications and consequences, are. Perhaps some, even many, can be eliminated altogether, and others used only when the probabilities are high that they will produce valuable results or outcomes. The consensus panels of the NIH, the American Medical Association's Diagnostic and Therapeutic Technology Assessment (DATTA)

Program, the *Medical Technology Assessment Directory* of the Institute of Medicine, and the Clinical Efficacy Reports of the American College of Physicians, for example, are useful and necessary.[49]

Yet there is no reason to think that they will, with some exceptions, meet the hope invested in them, or to think that they can by themselves transcend the human biases and values, the social and cultural forces and expectations, that are the social and political context of our national addiction to technological advancement.[50] Technology assessment is a movement that, in great part, itself threatens to become one more example of the touching faith in technical fixes for complex social problems that has long been a part of the American landscape. At bottom, the entire technology assessment movement lacks any overall perspective, or value framework, by which to make judgments on the moral or social worth or value of different technological goals. If we shared a consensus on the human good and human ends, technology assessment could be effective. Lacking that consensus, technology assessment can have little bite. It lacks real substance. All it can do, at its best, is develop some figures and projections, some more or less raw data on economic (and social) costs and benefits. It can assess the relative efficacy, and point out the economic consequences and implications of both old and new technologies. But it cannot by its purported value-neutral methods offer any help whatsoever in judging whether it would be justifiable to bear those consequences. It cannot quantify, or in any other way evaluate, the selection of appropriate goals for the use of a technology or determine what costs are humanly and societally *worth* bearing. Albert R. Jonsen has noted one striking way this deficiency manifests itself, in its failure to overcome "the role of rescue." By that he means the way in which a technology not otherwise cost effective gets used if it will save life. That means we are "unable to extend our felicific calculus to the very expensive technologies that will rescue the relatively few," which is just where we most need that calculus, of course.[51]

Technology assessment cannot, most critically, determine

whether and to what extent to make use of a technology that will give a mixed result, which is what most technologies do, particularly those still in a state of transition and continuing refinement. It takes a great deal of assessment and a working social and medical consensus to decide, say, that use of a technology is unnecessary, unsuccessful, unkind, unsafe, or unwise, to take some sensible standards proposed by Bryan Jennett.[52] Consider simply two of his criteria, *unkind* ("prolongs life of poor quality") and *unwise* ("diverts resources from other health care activities that would bring more benefits"). Each of them, to be meaningful, must embody a deep view of human welfare and happiness. Only rarely will the results of any assessment, using such criteria, be crisp and clear cut. They will ordinarily be contentious, and at least debatable. How are we to assess a technology that helps some but not all, and where we cannot clearly know in advance who those some are? Or a technology that provides a small benefit to a large number, but a benefit powerfully sought by them?

The answers to such questions cannot be given by the methods of technology assessment. They can only be supplied by the moral context and cultural setting in which the results of the assessment are deployed. If that setting cannot be changed—as is still typically the case—then those results can either be pushed aside or, by dint of passion and interests, be judged acceptable. Successful technologies will provide the hardest cases for evaluation. As Gregory de Lissovoy has nicely shown, "the typical new patient in the Medicare kidney disease program is older and sicker than in previous years" and, in the case of heart transplants, "the most significant revelation is that the 'acceptable' upper age limit for transplant candidates has increased rapidly."[53] Why is that? Because dialysis and transplantation are increasingly judged successful with sicker and older patients. Money aside, they seem to pass one common test of technology assessment: They work, at least in the judgment of those who can choose them—doctors and patients. At the same time, lacking any consensual criterion other than some kind of technological success as the standard for acceptable treatment, the number of users (and the cost) continues to climb.

The lack of a moral and evaluative foundation for making solid judgments about what would provide high-quality care, much less what would serve to limit the growing cost of such care, in the end renders technology assessment a weak tool by itself for making the hard choices. Even worse—as much present enthusiasm for its deployment suggests—it is looked upon as a way of avoiding unpleasant moral and political choices and thus diverts attention from the most difficult problems of resource allocation, those requiring a sacrifice of efficacious treatments.[54] Getting rid of ineffective technologies is thus only part of the problem, the morally and socially easy part (even if full of practical obstacles).

The most common and misguided assumption is that, if a technology is efficacious, particularly highly so, we should therefore use it—and we should therefore be able to afford it. Yet what expensive ineffective technologies have in common with expensive effective technologies is that they are both expensive. That the efficacious technology *is* effective does not, however, mean that it is any more *affordable* than the ineffective one. Efficacy and affordability are two entirely different matters, and their implicit conflation in much technology assessment promotion contributes enormously to the illusion that the key to cost containment lies in determining which technologies will be efficacious. This could well be called the *efficacy fallacy:* if it works, we should therefore be able to afford it.

The most important point to be kept in mind about the use of assessment of technology to increase efficiency is that the greatest long-term healthcare costs have come with the success, not the failure, of medicine. We of course need to know if a technology will fail. We need even more to know what its success will cost and will mean. The triumph of medicine—in extending life spans, in producing cures, in reducing morbidity, in providing effective rehabilitation from disability (but still never succeeding in doing more than delaying a final illness and death)—is what has, in the aggregate, driven up the costs. The pre–World War II medicine that was so inexpensive was also ineffective. The price of success of good medical care, of the achievements of medicine, is to make people want more successes, which will thereby raise their overall bill. "The cost of the health system," Dr. Maurice McGregor has written, "increases in proportion to the success of each technological innovation."[55] People are saved from one disease only to be put in a position to incur the costs of another disease and in general to be led by the power of technology to ever higher levels of desire and aspiration, to want cures for each succeeding illness. In his study of efforts to control the costs of hospital care, Dr. William Schwartz concluded that substantial short-term savings can be achieved, even $20 billion to $25 billion, but, "by the end of the decade, all of the saving from this policy would be exhausted." He concludes on a sober note, arguing that "the long-term control of the rate of increase in expenditures thus requires that we curb the development and diffusion of *clinically useful* technology."[56] It is success, not failure, that economically does us in.

A similar point can be made about the pursuit of research. In every field these days, and particularly before Congress, the case is made that a greater investment in research will eventually bring down the cost of healthcare. Just as the iron lung gave way to inexpensive polio vaccines, so too research will continue to find inexpensive ways to avoid the high cost of illness. As a vigorous and otherwise thoughtful examination of research possibilities to manage aging put it: "The means may be at hand to avert major diseases of aging and perhaps to intervene in aging itself, so that health and vigor are maintained longer, and disease and disability are reduced to a minimum prior to death."[57] "At hand"? That may be a perfectly true *theoretical* possibility (how could one *prove* otherwise?), but there is no certainty that it will come out that way and the evidence to date, in fact, is at best only fragmentary and suggestive in that direction, and offset by different evidence going in a contrary direction.

A common mistake in this respect is the expectation that, just as the infectious diseases that once took many lives (typhus, smallpox, yellow fever, and the like) came to be eradicated or controlled in inexpensive ways (vaccinations or antibiotics), the same pattern of success can be repeated with the present chronic illnesses (cancer, heart disease, stroke) and particularly the maladies of the old. History is expected to repeat itself. But in fact as people have lived longer, chronic illness has increased and continues to do so, and technology has heavily succeeded in keeping alive, at some cost, those whose death would have precluded the decline that has become increasingly attenuated, not reversed (even if not necessarily the oldest old, but those in somewhat younger age groups).[58]

As for the general possibility that a greater research investment will eventually lower healthcare costs, all evidence to date suggests just the opposite. Data provided by the National Institutes of Health are illuminating. (See Figure 2, p. 276.) Between 1979 and 1987, for example, there was a 180 percent increase in total health costs and an identical 180 percent increase in health research and development.[59] Research does not retard cost increases; research correlates with an increase in costs. As the very first figure in the annual *NIH Data Book* makes clear, the investment in research and the cost of care markedly parallel each other, rising at almost precisely identical rates for many decades now.[60]

The sustained growth of biomedical research since the Second World War has helped to stimulate public desires, even greater aspiration on the part of researchers, and the development of a variety of sub-industries and groups who benefit from the advancement of technology. If research was known to be an effective means of reducing costs, there would be very little incentive for industry, or the researchers themselves in some cases, to pursue it with their accustomed zeal. The fact of the matter is that, in medicine as in the rest of our contemporary life, technology opens up new possibilities, finds new ways to put people to work, provides for the production and development of new devices, and in general intensifies powerful forces of spending and consumption already present in the society. The promise of saving lives and improving health blesses those forces in an irresistible way.

The economic history of the healthcare system of the United States should be seen as a disturbing one for the cost-containment movement, which has failed to grasp the healthcare system's driving force. The system shows a constant escalation of costs, in great part because it has been stimulated by the desire for even better care, more choice, more profits, and higher returns for all. Neither technology assessment nor greater research nor pursuit of quality care at a low cost (or all of them together) are going to be sufficient to change the course of that history. Cost containment and greater efficiency are often offered as an alternative to unpleasant, undesirable rationing. The obvious difficulty with that position is that effective cost containment, of a kind yet to be seen in the United States, is nothing other than a form of rationing. If and when cost containment begins to take hold, it will be because of a tacit recognition of that reality, and because some basic values were changed to make it possible.

## FINDING A WAY OUT—THE COST OF CHOICE AND THE BURDEN OF MORTALITY

The ultimate problem behind the failure of cost containment and the quest for efficiency is an unwillingness to confront some disturbing implications of our highest ideals. We want to change the mechanics of the system rather than to examine the psychological, moral, and political assumptions that lie below it. The most fundamental of those assumptions is that cost containment can be made compatible with the preservation of choice and constantly enhanced quality, and can be made achievable with minimal government interference and regulation. Permeating everything is the ideal of meeting individual curative needs, needs ostensibly defined by the individual but actually also stimulated by the cultural backdrop of a love of expanding choice and technology innovation. A more ingenious method of thwarting efficiency and cost containment could hardly be imagined. If there is ever to be a way out of this situation—deeply a part of our national life—then we must look in two directions for new possibilities. One of these directions is the institutional, the other the moral and philosophical.

There are four unpleasant lessons to be learned at the institutional level if cost containment is to succeed: Government must be given a strong regulatory hand; there must be some form of universal healthcare coverage; freedom of choice must be limited; and technology assessment must be superintended by a willingness to apply strict standards of efficacy based on some substantive view of human well-being—and by a willingness to use these standards to reduce or eliminate the use of effective technologies when unaffordable, not just those that are ineffective or marginally effective. The necessity of a strong government hand is a conclusion I draw not from any theory about the value of government, much less governmental regulation, but from the universal experience of every other developed country in the world.[61] The willingness to accept regulation, and to live by it as a daily constraint, is the single thread that binds together all those countries that spend less on healthcare than the United States but achieve equally good, or often better, health outcomes, that is, rates of illness and death. Our lack of a unified system is a major source of our troubles, and a meaningful system for cost containment requires some form of central control (or centrally organized standards).

The lack of any intrinsic limits to health needs and the possibilities of medical progress can have only one meaning: If limits are to be set, they must be imposed from the outside and they must be imposed by political force. Otherwise, as we see in the United States, health "needs" take on a life of their own, constantly escalating. There can be relatively efficient or inefficient means of meeting individually defined health needs, and the same can be said for the pursuit of medical progress. But that is a narrow kind of efficiency, focusing on means and not on ends. If it is in the nature of the enterprise itself—because of its expansive goals—to constantly break boundaries, that form of efficiency will make a minor difference only. Only a strong governmental hand can contain the enterprise itself. None of the other actors will have a sufficiently strong incentive to do so.

To speak of the necessity of government regulation is, naturally, to accept the idea of an imposed limitation on choice; they cannot be separated. Patients have to be restricted in the kinds of choices they are given about their healthcare, physicians restricted in the diagnostic and therapeutic choices they are given about providing that care, and institutions restricted in the range of services they can provide and the ways in which they provide them. These limitations, moreover, must be instituted on a systemwide basis, so that a savings in one area is not offset by increases in other areas (as happened with the DRG effort).

I do not deny that there will be many losses, both personal and professional, in policies of that kind. It is thus important to be clear what the ultimate choice is: If it is necessary to control healthcare costs, and one is serious about that, then the clear historical record shows that it is naive to believe it can be done wholly by self-restraint on the part of individuals and private institutions. While controls may not be against their long-term interests (as I will argue in the next two chapters), controls will surely thwart their short-term desires and demands, which include seeking what they think they need in the ways they want to pursue it, a generalization as true about the patient seeking care as about the physician providing it. The serious question is not just whether restriction of choice is needed to effect cost containment (or incentives and disincentives which have that effect). It is also whether those restrictions can be developed in a way that makes societal sense while respecting the core of individual worth and dignity (which I will also explore in the next chapter).

Where will technology assessment fit into this necessary role of government and the restriction of choice? Despite all its shortcomings, some form of it will be needed.[62] But two points should be understood about meaningful technology assessment. The first is that it is a useless (and expensive) exercise unless there is a willingness to engage in prospective assessment before technologies are introduced, and to *force* a discontinuation of the use of those technologies that are ineffective or only marginally effective, or effective but too expensive to find social justification. There must also be a willingness to enforce a ban even when, as will often be the case, there will be a lack of full agreement about the assessment. The second is that there must be, to offset likely disagreements, a willingness to seek, and powerful pressure to achieve, some significant degree of social consensus on the moral, normative standards for effectiveness and efficacy. Beyond a point of sensible efforts at cost containment, claims of the legitimacy of different pluralistic standards will have to be rejected. To leave those standards to individual judgment is nothing less than to capitulate to the force that creates the need for cost containment in the first place—the desire for total private control and professional discretion. It is not that government control and a denial of liberty are patently good ways of gaining control of costs. They are not necessarily good at all. They are just necessary and unavoidable.

If a change in political direction will be required for serious cost containment, a still more difficult change in our way of thinking about illness and health is needed. There is a hard philosophical truth at which we have avoided looking, one that must be radically disquieting for any hopeful beliefs about the possibility of some ultimate efficiency. It is simply the burden of mortality: *Illness, decline, aging, and death can only be forestalled, kept at bay, never permanently vanquished.* Just as this burden works ultimately against the idea of meeting individual need, it works no less powerfully against controlling costs, at least if the goal is to simultaneously pursue unlimited medical progress *and* efficiency.

Consider the implications of the reality of mortality for cost containment. One implication is that, as the easier causes of disease and death are understood and managed, the costs of dealing with those that are more complex and intractable will and must grow, at least if we insist upon moving ahead with a continued high sense of urgency to find cures for those that remain. Efficiency can only be relative in that context and costs must increase. At the same time, as we well know, the price of the progress can be an increased prevalence of chronic illness, the result of slowing but not vanquishing decline and death.

## TWICE CURED, ONCE DEAD

Another, closely related implication is what I have come to think of as the "twice cured, once dead" phenomenon. A person saved from death at one time in his life is a person bound to die at some other time. Both incidents must be paid for, and both sets of costs need to be calculated to find the total societal costs of a lifetime of care for a person. We can in principle, and often in practice, bring down the costs of responding to life-threatening incidents. But we will still have to bear the (even reduced) costs of the illness we are trying to cure as well as, unfortunately (from an economic perspective), the costs of succeeding illnesses, those the patient can now live to incur because of our success in keeping him alive by earlier interventions. The well-known fact that a relatively small proportion of people, 10 percent, account for a significant proportion, 75 percent, of overall costs illustrates the problem perfectly.[63] Advanced medical care saves them from one incident or crisis after another; they neither die nor are fully cured (at least from their predisposition to become repeatedly sick). They are twice (or thrice) cured, but once dead.

Lewis Thomas's vision of an end to all halfway technologies, to be replaced by those that are both inexpensive and decisively effective, may only be the latest of modern medicine's myths. The problem is, as the psychiatrist Willard Gaylin has noted, that all technologies are halfway technologies if they do not cure aging, decline, and death, which none yet do or are likely to do.[64] This same reality puts the problem of preventive medicine (or health promotion, as it is now often called) into a new light as well. If its aim is an absolute saving of money, that may well be impossible: Illness is simply deferred and postponed, not eliminated altogether. People will die of something, and there is no guarantee that the illness they finally die of later in life will be less expensive than others earlier averted by successful health-promotion efforts (an issue to which I will return in Chapter 7). Just what exactly is the social or economic benefit of saving someone from death from heart disease in middle age (increasingly possible) only to have that person succumb to Alzheimer's disease in old age (increasingly likely)? Or to save a person from an early death from lung cancer (having successfully persuaded him or her to stop smoking) only to make possible a later death from stroke (or from, inevitably, *something*)?

These are not meant to be mischievous or morally insensitive questions, nor does asking them necessarily open the way (as some have objected to me) to a *reductio ad absurdum*—that it might be cheaper simply to let everyone die at birth. We do want to live, and it is worth a great deal of individual and social spending to make that possible. I only want to point out that the enterprise of healthcare has within it some inherent paradoxes and limitations, those that the mortality and finitude of the body impose. We can work against that limitation and beat back that finitude. But we cannot conquer them, and it will be our inability to do so that must remain a permanent obstacle to perfect efficiency in the pursuit of medical progress. Our problem, then, becomes one of great difficulty and delicacy. If we cannot finally overcome our mortality and if we also know (as we now do) that the cost of trying can grow increasingly high, then what would be reasonable goals for a healthcare system—reasonable in meeting the "needs" of individuals and the common health need of society as a whole, and reasonable in terms of managing our resources, resources that must be devoted to individual and social goods other than health? I have tried to show that our present system, focused on meeting individual curative needs and yet desperate for efficiency and cost containment, can only fail. I now want to offer an alternative.

# CHAPTER 4

# HEALTH AND THE COMMON GOOD: SETTING SOCIETAL PRIORITIES

The paradox of health is that it is both acutely personal and consummately public. Its personal side is evident. Our individual bodies become ill and are threatened with death. We get sick and die one by one. The pain and suffering that accompany illness are intensely private, directly known only to ourselves and by others only through our testimony. We never feel quite so alone, so isolated, as when we are ill; our pain, anxiety, and suffering turn us in upon ourselves. We alone can find meaning, or cause for despair, in the experience of sickness.

Yet health is no less public than private. Our illnesses affect the lives of those around us, sometimes because our disease is contagious, and sometimes because our private suffering can bring anguish to others and the need for their care. Whether we consider ourselves sick or well will to a considerable extent reflect our social definitions of health and illness. Whether we think our condition bearable or insupportable will manifest our beliefs about the relative acceptability of pain and suffering, usually culturally influenced. While we experience our suffering alone, the love and help of others can significantly lighten its burden.

Good health requires social networks and systems, whether they be for providing basic public health measures, for creating institutions to meet acute medical needs, for nursing and chronic-care needs, or for that kind of familial, institutional, or government support that cuts through all of those domains. In the face of the high costs of contemporary medicine, the individual is heavily dependent upon society for some form of third-party payment, private or public; the costs would otherwise be prohibitive. Society in turn is heavily dependent upon government, which subsidizes medical education and research, hospital construction, and long-term care facilities and provides an infrastructure of public health activities.

Illness itself is as much social as individual in its characteristics. We know, for instance, that the relative tolerability of illness for the individual will be much determined by the kind of care and support provided by others, and beyond that by the social meaning of a disease (compare AIDS with polio, for instance). We know also that illness is heavily determined by forces other than individual choice and behavior. Prenatal conditions, genetic predispositions, and environmental factors are obvious instances of that generalization. Even though poor personal behavior can be a significant cause of illness, we also know that social circumstances can be a major contributor to that supposed personal choice.

Here again we see the paradox. Though we suffer and die one by one, both health and healthcare are social phenomena, whether in those forces that bring poor health or those that help us overcome it. That it is individuals who have the poor health and suffer pain that only they can know directly should not distract our attention from the social contexts and determinants of all that affects health. A society that thinks of illness as simply an individual phenomenon, with an occasional public face, is already on the wrong track.[1]

What are we to make of the relationship between individual and social dimensions in the way we think about healthcare? The argument I want to make can be quickly stated. We have no lasting hope of devising a decent understanding of health—and thus of fashioning a viable healthcare system—unless we learn better how to attend to the social dimension of health, indeed unless we learn how to shift our priorities sharply in a societal direction. We have tried for many decades to meet individual curative needs, but we should now have discovered that medical progress has made that goal too open-ended, too limitless, to be any longer wholly plausible. We have also thought that the only real obstacles to meeting individual need are medical ignorance, which research can overcome, and wastefulness and poor quality, which a strong dose of efficiency can cure. That is a misplaced faith as well. Stimulated by mistaken goals and comforted by false hopes we have been left, despite efforts at reform, with a healthcare system whose state can only be likened to an explosion, driven relentlessly outward by the combined force of an aging population, technological progress, and a relentless public demand to meet ever-expanding individual needs.

We need instead a system that can find its own limits, that intensifies its force of progress inward, and that aspires for itself a responsible, not imperialistic, place in our common life. The key to that possibility is to switch our gaze and our thinking from the individual to the societal perspective. We will and must come back to the individual, but I want to argue for a different starting point, a fresh way into our problem of healthcare.

## FINDING THE PLACE OF HEALTH: INDIVIDUAL AND SOCIAL

The place to begin that effort—the only place it can begin—is by examining the place of health in human life and of the pursuit of health as part of a societal or communal way of life. We can ask some basic questions, and I will pose a few that are fundamental. Why is it that we as individuals want health, how much of it ought we to want, and what is the good it will bring us? Other questions are social. Just what is it that good health brings to a society and how much and what kind of it are necessary for a good society? What is the common good it will bring us, and what is the public interest that it serves? Yet if we can ask about the meaning and place of health from an individual and a societal perspective, we can hardly avoid noticing how inextricably related they are; the boundaries are not clear and the lines of influence are overlapping and interdependent. Our view of health affects the way we understand our private lives, just as it will influence the way we interpret our social and cultural way of life as a people. But how does our view of health affect our view of life, and how does our view of life affect our view of health?

That is an intimidating list of questions, and I phrased them in a way that would invite an effort to determine what, in actuality, we think. Yet we could approach them in a different way. What *ought* to be the way we understand such matters? Which interpretations of the relationship between health and human life will help us to find a *proper* and *sensible* and *reasonable* perspective, especially when we come to apply it to the fashioning of a healthcare system? I moved, with those questions, from the realm of description to that of moral substance—by the use of words like "ought," "proper," "sensible," and "reasonable." That is a move we find awkward in a pluralistic society, one wary about a common pursuit, much less common answers to questions of ultimate human goods, purposes, and goals. Because the pursuit of health, moreover, appears such an obviously good and clear goal, it has seemed unnecessary to probe too deeply. Yet they are the central and unavoidable questions and the ones we must talk about as a society if we are to have any hope of coping well and humanely with the allocation problem. They are, inescapably, matters of moral substance.

Where should we start in trying to answer such questions? I begin at the beginning: For what ought we to live? The principal goals of human life may be understood as twofold. We seek to understand what counts as the human good in general and what is good for us as persons in particular—we want to know who we are as individuals and what we are to make of ourselves for ourselves. We no less seek, psychologically and socially, to develop our capacities to love, to work, to think and feel, and to find our place within the communities of which we are a part. Our lives turn inward and they turn outward and we move back and forth between the private and the public spheres, the hidden life we spend with ourselves, the domestic life we spend with our family and friends, and the public lives we spend with others, either mere acquaintances or total strangers.

Why do we pursue good health? Because some degree of good health is a necessary condition for living with ourselves and living with others. Although it is perfectly possible to talk of health as a state of affairs in its own right—as bodily integrity, for instance, or a set of statistical norms (e.g., acceptable blood pressure)—if we ask what *good* the state of affairs is, why we should care about it one way or another, the answer is that health is a means to our other goals and purposes in life. It makes their realization possible, not wholly but importantly.

Good health in the absence of a sense of purpose or meaning in life can seem a worthless good. It will have value if purpose can be generated for the life it is meant to serve, and only then can it take its place as a valued means in achieving that purpose. Here we may recall the earlier discussion (Chapter 2) of individual needs. We have body needs because we want to live, psychological needs because we want to use our reason in managing our lives and our emotions in being at one with ourselves and others, and function needs because we want to act, to do things with and in the world. Yet, even saying that, health remains a means.[2] It does not give us our ends, does not tell us why we should want to live, or what we should use our reason for, or how we should feel, or what kinds of acts and functions are good and bad, right and wrong. Those are the deepest and most basic human questions, and good health provides us with not the faintest hint or clue about their answers. If we have good health, but have no answers to those questions, we are in deep trouble in our private lives. Our lives then have no meaning and that is the worst kind of death. Far better to have good answers and poor health.

Health may be understood as a means in two senses. Negatively, we seek good health to avoid pain and suffering, which in sufficient intensity can make life a misery and seem not worth living. Positively, we seek good health in order that we can effectively pursue our life goals. Poor health is a danger to that pursuit and death the ultimate threat. The particular type of life that we decide to pursue as individuals will of course make a difference in the way we understand health as a means. We would expect the athlete to seek different health goals than the desk worker. So also the way of life of a society will make an analogous difference. A technological society such as ours may seek different health goals than an agricultural society. To note such things is only to affirm that the notion of "good health" can have different senses and possibilities depending upon context and circumstance. It does not disturb the main point, however, that health is a means to our human good in general, and our personal ends in particular.

The relationship between health as a means to avoid pain and suffering and as a means to achieve some positive good is important to consider. A life devoted sheerly to the former goal would not only be one bound to frustration and ultimate failure, but it would also contribute to the shaping of a life both hypochondriacal and narcissistic. The notion that we can control life sufficiently well to gain only pleasure, and avoid pain, is alluring and widespread. There is no good reason, however, why we need to devise a healthcare system to help people live that way. On the contrary, since health is best understood as a means and not an end, it will not be surprising that we can as individuals often get by with less good, or ideal, health than we might like, and even on occasion less than what we reasonably need. It is a flexible and not fixed need. The force of habit and the power of adaptability allow us as human beings a remarkable range of response to and tolerance of illness. Life can go on, and often well enough, in the face of disability, chronic illness, pain, suffering, and even imminent death. We are remarkably resilient, flexible, tough, and enduring creatures. If we cannot have the health we want, we can often (not always, of course) learn how to do without it. We hold in constant tension, then, the dream of good health and a recognition that we can get by with something less, often much less.

We do not, of course, think about our individual health wholly apart from the society and the culture of which we are a part, however much our sense of good or bad health will seem intimately, inescapably personal. Society and culture provide us, among other things, with the values with which we judge the state of our health in comparison with others, our expectations about our health and what it is reasonable to hope (or not hope) for, the meaning and significance we bring to our illness, decline, and death, and our sense of the potentialities for improved health. None of these possibilities seems fixed by our human nature. One way or the other, it appears, people learn to adapt to the level of health available in their society, an adaptation that may blend elements of hope and resignation, aspiration and fatalism, acceptance and rage, meaning and despair. They have to live with what is available, and adapt their lives to it. They may hope for more, but they will if necessary settle for less.

This consideration is important to bear in mind as we move from a focus on individual health to that of the collective health of a society as a whole, and to devising a perspective on health as part of a way of life. But what is the proper place of the quest for health in devising a societal way of life? That question might equally well be posed another way: What societal way of life will most help us pursue sensible health goals? I have been critical of a way of life that simply says, as ours usually does, that it is not the business of society to openly discuss what is ultimately good or bad for individuals, that we should simply let them define their individual needs as they see fit and then bring science and commerce to bear in helping to achieve these needs. I have suggested that we cannot afford to seek the endless satisfaction of individual curative needs as defined by the possibilities of endless medical progress. But to reject that view is to reject in great part the way of life of which it is an expression. We must think differently, then, about the way of life in which healthcare is embedded, the meaning and value we attribute to health itself, and the relationship between individual and societal health.

# DEVISING A WAY OF LIFE

How might we think of the place of health in our way of life? We cannot ultimately meet the individual need for the cure of all illness and the staying of death. That notion has become all but meaningless, and it is hazardous to pursue. We need an alternative goal. The primary goal, the highest priority, of the health-care system as a curative effort should instead be that of fostering the common good and collective health of society, not the particularized good of individuals. The focus of concern with individuals (as I will develop later) should be that of care rather than cure—guaranteeing them decent and basic support in the face of illness and death, but not an unlimited effort to vanquish them. This would not by any means entail a displacement of concern for individual wants and perceived needs, but of redefining the needs to be met and giving them a different kind of place in our way of life.

By giving priority to societal health, I mean to suggest that health should be understood as a common benefit, something we need for our life together, not just one by one. We share in the good health of each other just as we are to some greater or lesser extent diminished as a people if illness is too common among us. Historically, the impact of plagues and epidemics gives us a vivid sense of what happens to all the institutions of a society when illness becomes a pervasive reality. Everything suffers—families, traditions, government—not simply individual people. It is important that this point be understood, for it would be all too easy to interpret the idea of a societal priority as making individual welfare irrelevant. Not at all. It is, instead, to say that a primary social good of a society is general good health. It serves the interests of all by making possible the functioning of its key institutions.

Here is the kind of question we should then ask: How much and what kind of health does a society *in general* need in order to accomplish its purposes as a society? A different, but significantly related, question is: How much and what kind of health does a society need in order to be a humane and decent community of human beings? The same level of health may not serve both purposes, and for just that reason it is important to separate the two questions. In the remainder of this chapter I want to suggest some ways of answering the first question, and then in the next chapter explore the second. Before going on, however, we must take another basic step. It is necessary to have some understanding and agreement about the main ends that a society ought to be pursuing. We require *some* consensus on proper ends, *some* sense of what constitutes our common good or public interest, so that we can then suitably relate the societal need for health to that good.

What are appropriate societal ends and how does good health as a means bear on them? The first, and many would argue most important, societal end is the maintenance in good working order of the political and legal systems. We are a democratic republic, one allowing citizens a voice in government, and we are a nation of law, requiring that everyone be afforded the protection of the law and recourse to law to redress grievances and correct injustices. We need, then, enough healthy citizens to ensure the robust functioning of the institutions that sustain those processes. The second end is that of a solid economic order, one that is conducive to national economic stability and strength. We need a substantial pool of people able to work well and hard, physically and mentally, to care for their own economic needs and, more generally, those of the society as a whole. A third end is that of national defense, the protection of the society against illegitimate threats to its sovereignty or important values and institutions. That requires a substantial pool of young people healthy enough to take up arms. A fourth end is the pursuit and transmission of knowledge and culture, both for economic purposes and for the flourishing of our institutions and traditions. We need a majority of people relatively free of want, emotionally stable, and satisfied with the rough contours of their life for that to be possible. We need children healthy enough to take advantage of educational opportunities. A fifth end is the maintenance of those institutions that provide the bonds and depth of a society: the family, charitable and philanthropic organizations, churches, and other voluntary associations and institutions, for example. We need people able to live and work together, able to form bonds of caring and helping.

I have not tried, with that list, to be comprehensive. There are other institutions, and sub-institutions, in our society that might be mentioned. The important point is that there be some clarity on the broad ends of society, and on the level of vitality of its major institutions necessary to achieve those ends. That provides us with an important starting point on the relationship of health and society.

I have placed the emphasis on the condition of institutions necessary for a viable society. There is, to be sure, an important sense in which societal ends of that kind have the good of individuals as an important outcome; societies do not exist over and above the individuals who make them up. Yet when we speak of the common ends of a people living together in a society—their shared desire for "life, liberty, and the pursuit of happiness"—and the institutions that help form and significantly constitute their shared life, we recognize that it is those institutions and their good order that are of fundamental importance to the public interest. How much and in exactly what ways is not germane to my concerns here. Nor do I, with that list of societal ends, make any pretense of offering a full theory of society or suggest any necessary order of priority. It is sufficient here only to note that the ends I have sketched would, I believe, command a wide consensus. Some immediate implications for the pursuit of health and the provision of healthcare are apparent:

*Not one* of these ends requires perfect or optimal health; they are compatible with a wide range of individual illness and disability.

*Not one* of them requires an unlimited pursuit of medical progress, much less the kind of unrelenting war against aging, decline, and death that our system seems eager to wage.

*Not one* of them requires a constantly growing proportion of the gross national product to be devoted to healthcare.

*Not one* of them requires the achievement of the WHO

definition of health, the meeting of all individual curative needs as defined by the progress of medicine, or attaining the highest-quality healthcare.

## HEALTH AS A MEANS, NOT AN END

Those conclusions, though they are only negative in their thrust, should help us put the supposed need for a constant improvement of health in a clearer light. We may want it, but we do not as a society necessarily need it. We can also better see the dangers of pursuing a goal of that kind. If we are not able to explicitly relate health as a means to specific and accepted societal ends other than health, then we open the way to allowing health inadvertently to become an end in itself. If that happens, we then run the further danger, already apparent, of making the pursuit of health itself a way of life. Lacking a sense of the proper ends of society, a sense of overall societal purpose and rationale, the pursuit of health becomes its own goal, one that focuses exclusively on individual health, one that feeds on itself, and one that knows no direction and no possible limits.[3] The pursuit of health then serves as a substitute for other, more important goals, and that is one way of understanding the large portion of the GNP given to expenditures on health. Health sought for its own sake, or because of the jobs or profits it produces, leads to a kind of personal and social madness. One can never get enough or be too safe. We will spend too much on health, be in a state of constant anxiety about mortality, and be endlessly distracted from thinking about the more important purposes and goals of life.

There is another implication in taking a societal perspective on healthcare. Even if it does not tell us exactly how to draw lines—where to say enough is enough—it helps us to know that we can find acceptable general grounds to stop or slow down our efforts to improve health. That is an important conclusion in a society prone to see the pursuit of improved health as an absolute and unlimited good, one that can legitimately overpower other needs. Health is not an absolute good. It is a high, but still relative, good. If it is impossible to meet all individual needs, and if decline and death are an intrinsic part of the human condition, then "good health" over a human lifetime must always be understood as the *comparative* absence of pain and suffering, illness and disease. We do not need all of our citizens in perfect health to mange our social institutions, and we do not as individuals need to be in perfect health ourselves to participate in those institutions.

We can then think of allocation strategies as aiming not to utterly eliminate the evils of illness and disability—impossible in any case—but to keep them at a level low enough that they do not pose a major obstacle to achieving the primary ends of society. The pursuit of health should not be seen as the pursuit of positive well-being, expansively pursued. Good health is not a substitute for a good life, and good health does not guarantee a good life. A good life, individually or societally, can be had without perfect health. Just as the person who lives in order to preserve health is a figure of just ridicule, so also should be a society that gives priority to a health policy that seeks perfection—the conquest of all illness and disease—as its only satisfactory resting place. Health can only be an imperfect and temporary good in human life, and good health once achieved can in any event only make possible other things.

But let us push a step further and focus more directly on the individual within his or her social context. We might think of the relationship between individual and society as constituting three realms. One of these is that of individuals in their social roles: as workers, or teachers, or government officials, for example. In those roles they work or cooperate with others to contribute to the functioning of the institutions of society, keeping them going and helping them flourish. Another set of relationships constitutes the interpersonal realm. Here we have our private or quasi-public groupings and relationships. We are friends, and colleagues, and spouses, and caregivers. A good part of the satisfaction of life lies in our relationships with other people, and some would say all of it. The final relationship, for so I will call it, is that of the individual with himself or herself: the way we understand our personal lives and purposes, the meaning we bring to bear on them, the way we develop our private hopes and interpretations of the world in which we live. It is in this realm that our uniqueness as individuals is most likely to be manifest. We can share it only in part, and our other relationships will probably never fully reflect the nuances of our individuality.

What should be the focus of the healthcare system? It is the first two realms, I contend, the social and the interpersonal, that are the appropriate focus of the healthcare system in its curative emphasis. It is the social aspects of the individual's life that the technological system can most appropriately minister to, not that which is private and unique in the life of the individual. When the healthcare system attempts to achieve "complete well-being" for the individual (as in the WHO definition of health) or to meet each individual curative need, necessarily unlimited in its possibilities, then it goes astray, beyond the bounds of the sensible and the reasonable, and beyond its reasonable interest in societal well-being. The goal of the healthcare system should be that of helping us to meet our occupational and social roles and duties while, at the same time, helping us to live effectively within the interpersonal sphere of our lives within communities. All of this is simply to say that, as a social system aiming at the cure of illness and the forestalling of death, the healthcare system should give priority (though not exclusivity) to its societal needs, not to the needs of individuals.

## HOW MUCH HEALTH DOES THE PUBLIC INTEREST REQUIRE?

I have argued that the pursuit of health is a social enterprise, that the good of society should take priority in the provision of curative medicine over the good of the individual in its pursuit. But that points us in a general direction only, even if a very different one than is customary. We will next need to have some agreement on the relative place and importance to be given healthcare needs in relationship to other societal needs; on the relative priority of different health needs; on the basis of moral claims to societal healthcare; on the limits of healthcare; and on the meaning of individual "need" within a larger vision of the place of health as a societal good.

There has been remarkably little discussion in this (or any other) society about the relative importance of health in comparison with other needs and goods. It should now become a central question. How might we best think about the place of the pursuit of health in the spectrum of societal needs? Let me begin to get at that question not with a theory, but by looking at our own situation. In the United States, the percentage of our gross national product spent on health has risen from 5.2 percent in 1960 to 11.5 percent in 1989. Is the reason for that an increase in death rates in our society during that period? No. On the contrary, health in that important respect improved significantly for all groups and all individuals during that time. (See Table 3, p. 270.) Death rates for every age group have declined enormously in recent years; between 1970 and 1984 that drop ranged from 13.2 percent for those over eighty-five to 49.3 percent for those under age one. The average age-adjusted decrease for all age groups was 23.6 percent.[4] Only in the case of blacks has there been a change in the wrong direction: From 1984 to 1986 average life expectancy for whites rose from 75.3 to 75.4 years, but it declined for blacks from 69.7 to 69.4 years (though this change was heavily related to murders and accidental deaths, not disease). Could the reason for the increase in health spending be that some catching up was necessary, as if in earlier eras the United States had badly fallen behind the health levels of other nations? That was not the case either. While not the highest in all categories, the health of Americans has long been high on the list of developed countries. While there has, to be sure, been an increase in chronic illness, that has come about because of the great improvement in reducing death rates; it is a function of the success of medicine, though it might be thought of as an odd kind of compliment.

By contrast, during the past fifteen years or so, there has been a widespread recognition of the deteriorating state of American education. The percentage of GNP devoted to it decreased from 6.4 percent in 1973 to 6.2 percent in 1986 (while the percentage going to health was almost doubling during the preceding two decades). Although the welfare system was showing signs of pathology in all directions, the percentage of GNP devoted to that set of problems remained virtually stagnant, even declining significantly in relationship to inflation for programs devoted to children. The percentage of children living in families below the poverty line increased significantly during the 1980s, from 13 percent to over 20 percent.[5] By any number of standards, life in the United States has not improved significantly for well over a decade. Decline or stagnation has been the more common economic and quality-of-life indicator—in education, housing, roads, heavy manufacturing, fighting crime, and research and development, for instance. Even though the defense budget is much criticized, it has remained in the 6 percent range for many years, virtually static. Only the proportion of resources going to healthcare has significantly increased, and with it there have been some tangible gains in health, but nowhere in proportion to the increased expenditures.

These data suggest that we should give a relatively less important place to health expenditures in the future. Health should not continue to have the privileged place it has gradually gained over the years. The recent growth of expenditures does not reflect corresponding health gains (suggesting that we have not invested the money all that well in any case) and, no less importantly, has occurred while the index of other societal goods has declined. Measured by the standard suggested earlier—the adequate functioning of our major social institutions—we already have a sufficient level of overall societal health, more than enough. Most of the growth in healthcare expenditures has come about because of the growth of public demand, a demand insulated for the most part by third-party payments, allowing individuals to pursue their individual health needs with little worry about the personal financial cost to themselves or the collective cost to society. It has also more fundamentally come about because we have let ourselves be seduced by the idea that, in healthcare, there is no such thing as enough.

Healthcare expenditures therefore remain an attractive category for spending. That is not so much because there is enthusiasm to add new entitlement programs (which there is not), but because some of those already in place—Medicare, for instance—have proven themselves resistant to significant cutbacks or even leveling off. Between healthcare as an employee benefit, and as government entitlement programs, the great majority of Americans have been covered for most of their major health problems. They have not on the whole been forced to ask about the social benefits of that coverage; it was sufficient that there was a supposed personal benefit for them. That pattern provides a poor direction for the future.

Will it be possible to achieve some consensus that healthcare should receive a lower social priority in the future, to gain a recognition that a steady growth in healthcare expenditures long ago in this country stopped producing commensurate societal (or even health) benefits? Necessity in the form of budget constraints will be one goad. But other considerations can be brought to bear. A starting point would be to promote recognition of an obvious point, that what is good (or seems good) for individuals is not necessarily good for society. None of us likes to hear that point; it assaults our self-esteem. That does not, unfortunately, make it a false statement. It is also becoming true, moreover, that an improved general health status of the populace promises to contribute comparatively little or nothing to overall national economic, social, and political strength (save for some deprived groups). That will of course be especially pronounced when other socially important institutions and programs are stagnating or deteriorating for lack of support and financing.

While the provision of healthcare has improved in many ways, that is not true of other institutions. The public schools have deteriorated and American students now fall below, often well below, international averages. The development of mathematicians and scientists, in particular, has declined along with them.[6] That is a terrible situation for a country that is heavily dependent upon scientific and engineering skills for its economic welfare. What is true of the school system is no less true of housing (where shortages of affordable housing are common in many parts of the country); industrial research and development (where we have badly fallen behind a number of other countries, most strikingly Japan); roads and highways (where deterioration of roads and bridges, or overcrowding, is now pandemic and will eventually require, by government estimates, $400 billion in expenditures); and parks and recreation (where the national park system is overcrowded, understaffed, and beset by aging facilities). I leave aside here the problem of day-care for working parents, grievously inadequate; the issue of urban ghettos with their large number of unemployed, often violent teenagers; the disposal of waste, nuclear and otherwise—and so on and so on.

In comparison with that wide range of problems, the health-care system is in excellent, even superb general shape. The longevity of Americans is the best in the entire history of the nation and, save for some special and minority groups, steadily improving. The average level of individual and societal health is *already* adequate to meet the general needs, and appropriate ends, of our society. It also appears, moreover, that once some general level of adequacy has been reached—the general conquest of infectious disease, for example—a society can flourish economically and culturally despite a great burden of illness (which will in any case be in great part the result of the greater longevity that has resulted from the successful conquest of the infectious diseases). While various studies of the economic "burden of illness" show the benefits that a decrease in illness could bring, they do not so well show the present benefits from an already high level of health.[7] Nor do they necessarily well reflect the way in which medical progress has defined as serious illness many conditions that might earlier simply have been tolerated.[8] There is no reason whatever to think that a poor *average* level of health at present lies behind our major social problems and needs (though it is clearly a source of problems for some subgroups). A large proportion of present health problems are problems on the ragged edge, whose cure or amelioration with present research priorities will simply push that edge somewhere else, a situation particularly true with the health of the elderly.

To suggest that we may already be reasonably well off, as individuals and as a society, may seem a jarring suggestion. It means, at the least, that it is unimportant that we are not necessarily "the best" any longer. There is no reason to think of health as some kind of competitive international game that we must at all costs win. A decent healthcare system, even if not the best, can be perfectly sufficient. It means also that we need not zealously pursue constant general improvement in the system. We can try to meet other societal needs first, changing our priorities for a time.

Yet if we come to accept that kind of a more modest standard—sufficiency, not perfection—how are we to interpret and accept an obvious reality, that all about us are people dying prematurely, or living lives blighted by illness or disability, or burdened by neurosis or depression? That is true enough, even though many conditions are of the ragged-edge kind; they will *always* be there in one form or another, no matter how far medical progress goes, and many precisely because medical progress moves on. The final answer to the question, however, is that the economic and social costs of trying to rid our society of those terrible illnesses eventually become simply too great, achievable only at the unacceptable cost of doing damage to much else of great importance. We cannot have everything we want. To attempt to eliminate all suffering in one part of our lives is to court the unavoidable likelihood that we will increase it in other parts. Yet even if we must at some point accept this limitation, and tolerate continued illness and suffering, there is a high general level of health. Most of us now have a good chance of dying in old age and already some 70 percent die beyond the age of sixty-five. The triumphs of medicine are far advanced, even though they could go much farther, to infinity. It is our capacity to enjoy, and profit from, and economically afford those triumphs that must stop short of that possibility.

What if we had adopted the stance I am suggesting fifty years ago? Think of all the progress we would have forgone, the lives that might not have been saved had a more relaxed, less vigorous attitude about medical advancement been dominant. This is a common response to any hint that we might slow down the war against death and disease. But it risks two errors. The first is to think that what was appropriate in the past remains equally appropriate in the present. Precisely because we made those past advances, we can now afford to think about changing our priorities; we are now far better off. The second error is to believe that the future must always repeat the past, that because we were successful earlier with one group of diseases, we will be equally successful with another. Some fifty years ago infectious disease was still a powerful force, and research and clinical ingenuity all but vanquished them (although, as with AIDS, new ones can still appear). We have now, in general, however, entered the era of chronic disease and illness as well as conditions associated with advanced old age, and they are proving far more resistant to conquest. There is no special reason to believe they can be vanquished, and certainly not as decisively as, say, yellow fever or smallpox; and surely not as inexpensively.

There is also a more probing, and probably discomforting, question we might ask. What special reason is there to think that further health progress will *greatly* enhance societal happiness or welfare—or that a forgoing of the kind of obsession with health and medical progress that has been the mark of recent decades will do us as a society *significant* harm? There is little reason to think that either will be true. We are already feeding more our hopes and desires than tending to important and enduring needs. The debate about rationing and allocation, about setting limits, will be a far more sensible one if we keep in mind how well off in general we are. We should not be complacent about a number of special unmet needs in our society, both individually and collectively. But we can be satisfied with the average level of health. It allows us to carry out quite adequately the main functions of our society.

Yet if that is the case, why should special efforts be devoted to those groups that fall well below the norm? One obvious reason is that the economic burden of the healthcare system is in fact greatly exacerbated by the problems of those groups. Their health is worse, their medical crises more common, and their costs disproportionate to their numbers. Poverty, lack of education, and a disrupted social and family life are major correlates of poor health. Another reason is that of equity. They should have the same opportunities as a group open to those already well off. There can be no good reason to exclude or neglect them. The healthcare system should be expressive of the solidarity of the community in the face of illness, suffering, and pain. While it will not be possible or sensible to meet every individual curative need, to exclude whole groups from attainable and reasonable goals already achieved by others violates justice and common sense. It deprives people of goods that, by virtue of their citizenship, they have helped make possible. Even a modest sense of realism, moreover, should also make us recognize that most serious health problems spill out, so to speak, into the street. They do so by way of the spread of infection, the special social pathologies that illnesses of poverty can generate, and by the demand placed upon public services, even if too late and too poor to do much good (and perhaps especially then). One way or another the problems of the worst-off become the problems of all. That is another sense in which illness and disease are social realities, not just the fate of individuals.

I have not yet given a direct answer to the question of exactly what priority healthcare should have among all of the various needs of society. I have only suggested that, in the future, it should have a lower status than has been the case for some decades now. It should not be allowed to overshadow or trump those other needs. It makes no sense to have the health domain increase its share of GNP while so many other societal needs are going unmet and so many other basic institutions are displaying gross deterioration. But that situation does suggest one standard for setting priorities. There should, at a minimum, no longer be any assumption that health needs are, by definition, more important than other needs, or that they justify a share of the GNP well out of line with other societal expenditures. That day has long passed. A second standard suggests itself as well. In comparing a possible investment in education, or roads, or parks, or health, which is likely to produce the greatest long-term societal gain for overall economic and social benefits? One can well ask also, in that context, whether an investment in those other areas would be likely to produce some direct or indirect health benefits as well. If so, that increases their claim. But even if they did not, they might still better promote future societal strength than a health expenditure. That would certainly seem true at this point in history for education, which has declined too far and for too long.

## WHAT IS A SUFFICIENT LEVEL OF SOCIETAL HEALTH?

Can we, however, go further than casual random remarks, reflections, and assertions. The late theologian Paul Ramsey once wrote that the comparison of health and other goods in a pluralistic society for the purpose of making allocation decisions is "almost, if not altogether, incorrigible to moral reasoning."[9] It is our misfortune that, incorrigible or not, we must find a way to cope with it; and, though contentious, it may not be as impossible an issue as he assumed. We must now decide in at least some rough fashion how large a place to give to meeting health needs and claims in the years ahead. That can no longer be left purely to chance or the random play of claimed individual needs or insistent interest groups. It is doubtless correct to say that the ultimate decision about the allocation of societal resources among a wide range of needs must be political. We must, that is, make a collective decision through our political process, in light of our personal and political values, about how we want to deploy our common resources. But if that process is to have any coherence and substance, it will be necessary to give it some content. What should we be thinking and talking about in the political arena, and in our own minds, and what is at stake?

Two approaches are possible. We can look at the problem of allocating resources to healthcare as an economic issue, asking whether, and in what sense, healthcare is a comparatively good investment of our money as a society. We can also ask, from a perspective of the kind of society we want, whether and to what extent a heavy investment in healthcare makes sense in relationship to other goods that should be part of that society. These two approaches can easily converge, but it is helpful to first look at them separately.

If we look upon an investment in healthcare as an economic issue, there is patently much to be said for it. It helps to cure illness and hold off death, goals greatly prized by most people and beneficial to society. It provides employment for a large number of people and, over the past few decades, has been a particularly valuable source of employment for minority groups. Hospitals and other health facilities are often the largest employers in many communities. The health industry also purchases many items of value: buildings, machines, equipment, supplies of one kind or another. Biomedical research not only contributes to health, but also has environmental, agricultural, and other benefits (especially through recombinant DNA research). The stimulation of technological developments creates devices, equipment, and drugs that can be sold abroad and, at the same time, provides additional forms of stimulation to technological innovation, of use outside of medicine.

But are not health expenditures essentially "consumption" expenditures, that is, more a way of spending money than generating new sources of income and societal wealth? There seems no decisive economic answer to that question. Biomedical research and technological development, as well as the manufacturing of many healthcare items, can count as productive, income-generating expenditures; and helping people to stay well, or curing them of their illnesses, makes a contribution to worker productivity. Yet many expenditures in the name of health do not generate wealth, but dissipate it. Large numbers of people are not made more productive by healthcare, and many people in their illness or dying consume large, and often fruitless, amounts of healthcare. Part of the problem here is that of determining whether, and in what ways, healthcare expenditures are economically efficient. There is clearly great variation in that respect, but one economic fact stands out in American healthcare: We spend significantly more on healthcare that any other nation, but do not have better outcomes as a result. Many nations do just as well by every significant index—especially morbidity and mortality rates— at much lower cost.

This reality is important in helping to judge one common argument about the healthcare system, its ability to generate jobs. If healthcare is a potent source of employment, particularly for minority and other groups, is that not in itself a strong argument in its favor? The economist Uwe Reinhardt has shown the mistake in that way of thinking. He notes that between 1981 and 1987, there was a total increase in American jobs of 13.3 percent; this figure embraced a 5.4 percent drop in manufacturing jobs and a 26.6 percent increase in healthcare jobs.[10] But with this drop in manufacturing jobs went a decrease in our national export potential (despite some medical technology exports), with consequent damage to our balance of payments. Moreover, as Reinhardt argues, "although it is tempting to justify expenditures by the jobs they create, any country run for long on this principle will inevitably end up with a second-rate economy. . . . To justify added health expenditures chiefly with appeal to the jobs they sustain should be beneath the dignity of a proud industry. It is an argument for losers."[11] The only proper justification for expenditure is that of the "social values of the services it produces," and, from that perspective, we are forced into the even more difficult realm of deciding what it is that we should want as a society, what it is that we should consider of comparatively high or low social value as an expenditure.[12]

Lester Thurow, for one, has contended that, because of a

diminishment in American productivity since 1965, we cannot afford the kinds of healthcare expenditures that might have been possible if it had remained high. Our educational attainments during this same period have fallen behind those of other developed countries, as have our research and development investments more generally. "Simply because of the size and growth of spending on health care," he writes, "resources that would otherwise be spent on health care will have to be diverted to solve some of these problems. The United States cannot maintain the present rate of growth in healthcare spending while simultaneously restoring productivity growth and increasing international competitiveness."[13] Stuart Altman has made an analogous point. Noting that predictions of a collapse of the healthcare system in the face of rising expenditures have not materialized, he notes nonetheless that it "continues to prosper at the expense of other needed federal services. . . . Our gross national product represents the total capacity of our country to purchase needed goods and services. When we double the amount spent on healthcare, there are fewer resources available for other needs."[14]

Herbert Stein, former chairman of the Council of Economic Advisors, has helped to bring the points made by Thurow and Altman into even sharper focus. Noting that the most dramatic change in the GNP in recent years is the reduction of investments owned by Americans (from 20.1 percent of GNP in 1973 to 14.3 percent in 1986), he points out that the investment decline was marked by a parallel increase in the amount going to consumption. Of that amount, "almost two-thirds of the increased share of consumption in the GNP took the form of an increased share of expenditures for health care."[15] By contrast, expenditures for education, for defense, and for consumption by the poor have remained relatively static. Stein's point is to argue that "budget decisions—about spending, taxing, and borrowing— should be the instruments of explicit decisions about national objectives and priorities in the use of national output and not ends in themselves."[16] We should, that is, ask about the relative value of healthcare in light of our "national objectives and priorities," an effort we have in fact not made in many decades. We have simply assumed that more and more healthcare is a good to be pursued. We should now be putting to one side that assumption and freshly locating the kind and amount of health-care expenditures among our appropriate priorities.

There cannot be a straight *economic* answer to the question of the amount of healthcare spending that is appropriate. If anything emerges from the effort of economists in trying to answer this question, it is that it is not only an economic issue. "Health-care costs," Thurow has written, "are being treated as if they were largely an economic problem, but they are not. To be solved, they will have to be treated as an ethical problem."[17] This perspective is consistent with that of Stein, in his emphasis on determining national priorities, and with the one I have advanced in arguing that or deepest problem is that of deter-mining the place health should have in our way of life. To take this approach is not to deny the value of a more conventional economic viewpoint, that of the value we are receiving for the investment we make in healthcare. At what point do we reach a marginal gain, such that we would make a better investment elsewhere?[18] But the problem in trying to answer that kind of standard economic question is that we cannot do so without some larger framework of ethical values and thoughtful national priorities.

To see if we can find a way through that maze, I want to propose some general principles, of a kind designed to frame and bring order to our thinking, not to provide us with automatic answers. The principles are these: (1) A society will have a sufficient level of health when an absence of good health does not account for a deficiency in the functioning of its major social institutions, and when the great majority of it citizens are healthy enough to carry out their characteristic social roles in the society, and (2) a society will have spent enough on healthcare when, after a full accounting, it judges that the resources it devotes to health are not being harmfully diverted from other important societal needs, and that the money that is spent on healthcare will not have damaging long-term consequences. I will call these the principles of "sufficiency" and "full accounting."

## The Principle of Sufficiency

What would it mean to assert that a society has a sufficient level of health? This principle is meant first to alert a society to the possibility or likelihood that further general improvement in personal healthcare, especially the cure of illness, might make little or no additional contribution to the overall welfare of society, however beneficial to some or many individuals.[19] If health is understood as a means, then it may well be that a level of health that falls short, even well short, of individual aspirations, or even societal aspirations, may nonetheless be perfectly adequate to meet the central needs and functions of the society. It is not evident, for example, that a general increase in average life expectancy (from, say, the present seventy-five years to eighty-five) would make any significant contribution to the overall welfare of our society. Some might aspire to a goal of that kind, but it should be evident that we can have a perfectly functional, decent society without it.

The principle of sufficiency, however, should be understood to refer only to overall averages and levels of health. There will always be, so to speak, a ragged edge of general sufficiency; that is also unavoidable. The principle of sufficiency should in addition encompass a way of recognizing the status and needs of groups that fall well below the general average; their health is not sufficient and should be improved. The appropriate social priority would be to concentrate on those groups whose inadequate health status impedes their participation in the life of the society.

Let me try, however, to be even more specific. The principle of sufficiency requires a number of determinations:

*Determining an adequate level of societal health in general, sufficient to carry out the other aims of the society.* There exist at present no generally accepted standards for determining when a society has in general reached an adequate or sufficient level of health.

International rankings of national statistics on general and infant mortality are commonly used as one way of measuring the adequacy of a country's medical effort or success, but they provide no measure of what, absolutely taken, counts as adequate or sufficient. The most pertinent societal test is whether, and to what extent, poor health accounts for failures and deficiencies in the major social institutions of a society. Is the political or economic sphere weakened because of poor general health? Is family life in general crippled by ill health? In the case of the United States, at any rate, I believe the answer to such questions would be no. Whatever the shortcomings of our social institutions, the poor health of their participants is not the cause. Has anyone seriously suggested that poor health is the reason we no longer compete well with the Japanese, or that it explains our children's inadequate grasp of science and mathematics?

The following kinds of standards could be refined to provide a measure of sufficiency:

A *general* test: The health of a population in general is sufficiently good when a great majority (four-fifths or more) can carry out a normal range of social functions and enjoy a normal range of interpersonal relationships. Is this not an arbitrary standard? Yes, in the sense that others might propose 85 or 95 percent as the standard (which I would think too high). But it is not arbitrary in a capricious way. It looks to our present level of societal functioning, and notes that our political, economic, social, and voluntary institutions are functioning adequately well; and, where they are not doing so (e.g., international economic competition), it is not poor health that is the explanation. All policy standards will in some sense be arbitrary (why a speed limit of sixty-five rather than sixty-four?). The pertinent question is whether it is a *reasonable* standard, and I only want to suggest that "four-fifths or more" is reasonable, neither too high nor too low.

A more *specific* test, using an adaptation of the idea of a "normal opportunity range" for each age group as formulated by Norman Daniels: The health of children is sufficient when the vast majority are healthy enough to receive an education and to have their ordinary physical and mental developmental needs met; the health of adults in midlife is adequate when the great majority are able to work, to carry out an ordinary range of domestic duties, and to engage in community activities; and the health of the elderly is adequate when a large majority are able to live out an adequate biographical life span (late seventies or early eighties) and are able to carry out interpersonal and community activities of a common type. I suggest these standards not by way of making a precise determination, but only to observe that standards *of this kind,* and *in this range,* are what we should be looking for. The worst kind of standard would be one which demanded perfection as its test—for example, 99.9 percent of children meeting the standards noted above. Precisely that kind of perfectionism is what drives up the cost of care while not necessarily, at the margin, improving our common life.

*Determining where subgroups of the population fail to meet those standards and what needs to be done to raise their health level.* Various subgroups within the population will fall below the general average, and efforts should be made to identify their general needs and what can be done to meet them. There are always going to be some individuals who will fall well below the general norm, and whose needs could not feasibly be met because of the ragged-edge problem. The general effort should fall on improving the condition of the group (e.g., socioeconomic) of which they are a part, not on trying to meet the individual needs of every member of the group. To attempt the latter would involve the conflict, discussed earlier, of trying to meet every individual curative need, with all its attendant difficulties. No less importantly, many of the health problems of disadvantaged groups stem from social and environmental causes. At some point, it makes far more sense to go after those causes than to use healthcare to remedy after the fact more systemic problems.

*Determining an appropriate balance between the collective desire for better average health and the other needs and possibilities of the society.* There is every likelihood that, however actually adequate the general health of a society, there will be a desire for an even higher standard. That has been the history of medical progress and public attitudes, powerfully abetted by the ordinarily valid belief of scientists that they can, in fact, effect improvement if given sufficient resources. That there will always be cases along the ragged edge also means that some people will not have the health benefits that others have, and there will be social and moral pressures to lessen that disparity. Both a general desire for better health—regardless of how good the present health already is—and pressures to eliminate the ragged edges, then, will place constant pressure on the healthcare system.

The only effective way to cope with those pressures is by keeping before the public eye the needs of other sectors and aspects of the society. A society with ever-improving health but inadequate parks and schools will not be a well-functioning society. Healthy but unemployed people will not find their lives satisfactory nor will the economy be in good shape if unemployment is too high. We lack as a society a good sense of the proper balance among the various needs of society, some kind of integrated and coherent picture with which to work in public policy. It is not too soon to begin attempting to develop one, particularly in order that the demand for better health, usually insistent, is not allowed to increase its already undue power.

## The Principle of Full Accounting

This principle is meant to serve as a cross-check on the idea of sufficiency. It should lead us to look for an answer to two questions: How much money should we spend on health, and, in our present and proposed spending on health, have we taken account of the full social (as distinguished from economic) costs that are entailed? To ask how much we should spend on health is nothing other than another, though different, way of asking what we take to be a sufficient level of health. But the difference is that here we need to ask a kind of balancing question: Are we spending a sufficient amount on health to achieve an adequate level of societal health while, at the same time, not spending so much on health that, inadvertently or otherwise, we are neglecting other important societal needs?

Our goal here should be to take a comprehensive look at the needs of the society as a whole, seeking a balance that is coherent and reasonable, taking account of both short- and long-term requirements and aspirations. A "full accounting" is thus one that tries, however hard the exercise, to account for the full range of social needs, not just health needs. Our interest-group politics, our penchant for short-term solutions, our lack of central planning, our wariness about grandiose notions of the human good and the public interest all work against such a full accounting. Our unwillingness to accept the reality of disease and death, only delayed and never vanquished, also works against it. Yet an effort at such a accounting is unavoidable if we are to deal with the question of sufficiency. If we do not deal with it, then the power of health demands is all too likely to put other societal needs in the shadows; health needs have an immediacy and insistence more potent than other needs, even if the latter are just as important.

There is another important sense of "full accounting." In trying to determine what we should spend on health, we need to have some feel for what the full bill over the long term will be. The present method of accounting is usually short term: What will it cost us to save a patient from this disease at this time and with what benefit, or what will it cost us now to carry out the research that will make it possible to save some other patient in the future? Yet a method of full accounting would want to know not only the cost of saving the patient from this disease now, but also the cost of paying for the—inevitable—later disease that will finally kill the patient. (See Tables 1, 5, and 6, pp. 268, 272, and 273.) While we may not know what that disease will be, we know that there will be *some* disease or condition that will, and must, kill him, and perhaps also some nonlethal condition that will require expensive and extended ministrations as well. We have to find a way for that full life-course reality to be part of our thinking. When we find a cure for a disease that might otherwise have killed a patient, we have to pay for the research and therapy to deal with that disease as well as the other diseases that we have not been able to control and which will ultimately, as the successor diseases, mean the end of the patient; and if we deal with that disease, there will be still another to take its place, and still another after that. There is now, and always will be, the ragged edge.

That is the point of saying that all technologies are halfway technologies: Death finally wins, and it will not be denied its economic cost any more than it will be denied its cost to life. We have yet to engage, for instance, in the full accounting necessary to understand what the transformation of old age has meant, particularly that part which has kept more people alive longer but which has seen a rise in chronic illness and an extending of the process of dying over a longer and longer period. We can no longer escape that kind of accounting. It is part of the economic and social reality of the success of medicine. Even if it is plausible that there may someday be a significant compression of morbidity prior to death, we should not base our present policy calculations on an assumption that *will* and *must* happen. Until the evidence is solid and sustained, we should work with present patterns and with projections based upon them (this issue is discussed further in Chapter 6).

How far out into the future should our "full accounting" go? I have no precise answer to that question, but at the least a span of two or three generations would seem necessary; that falls in the range of the foreseeable future. As Phillip Longman has noted, "Since the beginning of modern medicine, each succeeding generation has invested massively in researching and developing new medical technology. But such investments are never matched with reserves designed to pay for the cost of whatever new medical knowledge comes as a result. For this reason alone, the financing of healthcare becomes ever more problematic, with each new generation inheriting valuable new medical techniques but no dedicated capital to pay for their use."[20]

We are only now, for instance, beginning to see the full consequences for old age and its place in society of the successful introduction of routine immunization and antibiotics into healthcare many decades ago. That has increased life expectancies in general, and the life of those beyond eighty-five in particular. Or who could have guessed that the artificial respirator, which came into widespread hospital use only in the 1960s, would eventually move as it has now done to the home and there, at great financial and emotional cost yet to be fully determined, be used to keep children alive—children who will, assuming they survive the condition that creates the need for a respirator, die of some other condition eventually? Perhaps no one could have guessed that a shift to the home would happen, but the cumulative experience of many such technological developments and their unforeseen consequences means that we can increasingly make educated guesses about the future. Ignorance of the future is less and less an acceptable excuse for not taking it into account. It is just hard, not impossible, to do so.[21]

A *full* "full accounting" would have to begin with the cost of research to cope with a disease, and then move to its clinical introduction, and then to the cost of its successful implementation and (typically) widened use once deployed—and then, and only then, can we begin to see what the costs will, in the long run, be. To that we must add the related economic and social costs beyond those that are narrowly medical—for instance, the home-care costs of those whose lives are saved by curative medicine but who require long-term additional care as a consequence. To be sure, we will not be able to calculate those costs accurately. We do not have to—rough estimates will do. It is the exercise of reminding ourselves forcefully that there will *be* costs—and of the prospects that they *could* be insupportable—which will bring to the healthcare enterprise a needed imagination about the future and a necessary caution about what it may mean. The goal is to bring sobriety to our curative and technological enthusiasms, and that is a valuable way to do so.

# CHAPTER 5

# HEALTH AND THE INDIVIDUAL GOOD: THE PRIMACY OF CARING

The first step in thinking about healthcare is to determine the place of health among the full range of human and social needs. I have proposed some ways of making such a determination, and I have also argued that achieving an adequate level of societal health should take priority over meeting individual curative needs. Once we have done that, we are then confronted with taking the next step, no less complex: How can we decide which of the many, seemingly innumerable, illnesses and threats to health are more or less pressing? I will approach that question from two very different directions, first from the perspective of the overall welfare of society, developed in the preceding chapter, and then from the perspective of the individual. A decent and humane system—not merely a functionally effective one—must find a good equilibrium between a focus on societal requirements and a focus on individual well-being.

In thinking about health priorities, we would do well to remind ourselves of a point long made, well supported, and yet routinely neglected: The most important health gains up until very recently were those that came from aiming at the health of groups, not that of individuals.[1] The great historical improvements in life expectancy, from the seventeenth through the early-twentieth centuries, first came about as a result of better nutrition, sanitation, and general living conditions. With this phase was born the idea of public health and preventive medicine. I will call that the "first phase." The next most important set of gains, from the late-nineteenth through the mid-twentieth centuries, came about with the virtual conquest of infectious disease by means of vaccinations and antibiotics. This can be called the "second phase." Thereafter, as we have come to know, other improvements—surgical techniques, intensive care units, improved rehabilitation, organ transplants—have made some contribution. But this, the "third phase," has been accompanied by an increase in chronic disease and illness, particularly accompanying longer life expectancies: Cancer, heart disease, stroke, and the various dementias are the obvious examples of that.[2] Combined with an aging population, this last cluster of conditions does not promise to give way to rapid solutions. Since they are also predominantly conditions associated with aging, they will in any case almost certainly give way to replacement illnesses, that is, to other diseases, possibly chronic also, that will in turn become the successor marks of old age.

The success of those first two phases and our difficulty with the third suggest some important lessons, of direct bearing on the case for societal priorities. One of them is that healthcare directed toward the welfare of large groups at risk from common, pervasive, and relatively controllable health threats still remains the most effective and relatively inexpensive kind. A healthy environment, including the provision of sanitation and a good diet, makes the most important contribution to the good health of individuals. It is the kind of contribution, moreover, that is not addressed to the uniqueness and idiosyncrasies of individuals, but to their common features. Preventive medicine has the same feature: It is directed in general to that which promotes health for everyone, not for those at risk from some specific ailment. The techniques of the second phase— childhood immunization, on the one hand, and the use of antibiotics to cope with infections, on the other—turn out to have the same characteristics. They are directed to generic health hazards to which we are all comparatively subject, not to those less common, more idiosyncratic conditions not well or fully addressed by general public health measures or social and environmental responses.

## OUR COMMON CLAIM TO HEALTHCARE

The health hazards that have been so effectively dealt with by such means all spring, as a rough generalization, from external, exogenous threats and conditions—for example, environment, diet, life-style, hostile bacteria and viruses. They affect all individuals in relatively similar ways and pose comparable hazards to all individuals. The difficulties that we face, by contrast, with the chronic illnesses that now dominate healthcare—schizophrenia, Alzheimer's, cancer, heart disease, stroke, multi-organ failure—are in many important respects different. While it is true that we will not know in advance those to which we might personally be predisposed or vulnerable, they are not a general threat to all individuals, but threats much conditioned by genetic and other individually unique features. Many of them, most importantly, correlate heavily though not exclusively with aging. Our success in keeping people alive through their childhood and into their adult years means an increased risk for the chronic illnesses of later life.

What are the possible policy implications of that historical trend? Perhaps simple and ultimately inexpensive treatments (or prevention regimens) will someday be found for those diseases and conditions that most characteristically pick on individuals in their individuality. That is possible. Yet to make that kind of hope the foundation of policy and spending—to act and spend *as if* it must happen—is exceedingly unwise. It is a mistake to assume that the kinds of successes characteristic of earlier medical history will necessarily be repeated in the future. That so many of the most difficult conditions are associated with aging means also that, given human nature itself, the ragged edge of

aging will most likely *always* and *necessarily* generate new debilitating and lethal conditions to replace those earlier reduced or
eradicated. Even if, under the most optimistic possibility, there
is an eventual "compression of morbidity" (a shorter period of
illness prior to death in old age), their could still be frantic efforts
at that diminishing ragged edge to extend life and defeat death.
In any event, death always wins. To constantly invoke the
success of the past to justify research on the remaining health
agenda is not only costly, but increasingly so. There is also no
certain likelihood, much less guarantee, of success. The reality
of aging makes it certain, in fact, that it must sooner or later fail
in some fundamental ways.

What can we conclude? When we look at healthcare from
the perspective I have sketched here, a number of conclusions
can be drawn. The first is that the greatest benefit the healthcare
system can bestow is to focus its efforts on those approaches that
historically constituted what I have called the first two phases.
That means focusing on the population as a whole, not beginning with the special needs of individuals.

The second conclusion is that the system promotes the
greatest societal benefit by that focus at the lowest possible cost
per person. A healthcare system that provided *nothing* other
than sanitation, good food, a decently clean environment, childhood immunization, antibiotics, and trauma care would already
have done enough to assure that the majority of its citizens could
carry out their societal roles. The more the system attends to
individual needs not met by basic public health measures and
primary healthcare, the more it guarantees an ever-larger
agenda and ever-higher costs, and especially as the curative
research agenda gravitates, as it has, to conditions affecting the
individual lives of the elderly.[3] A society may move on beyond
that point, but there is no compelling reason to think it must do
so. A society cannot be said to owe its citizens the pursuit of
every medical possibility to meet every curative need, much less
when the possibilities of doing so are endless.[4]

The third conclusion is that it is much easier to morally
justify, and even demand, a strong societal role in providing that

kind of basic care. It benefits in principle everyone more or less equally, in much the same way as do fire and police protection and national defense. It has the supreme advantage that it provides a very general benefit, one in itself sufficient to meet the most important societal need for health, and it admits of limits, for we already can, at a reasonable and circumscribed cost, provide that level of healthcare without inherently limitless expenditures—particularly if we accept the fact that, while it will not achieve good health for all, it will achieve good health for a sufficient number to carry out the main functions of society. Exactly the opposite is true in the quest to meet individual curative need. It will not be possible for us to meet such need, no matter how hard we try or how far research advances, or to pay the costs of such a crusade, one ever doomed to fail on one ragged edge or another. But we can, as individuals, make a solid claim for a healthcare system that provides for the general health of society, of which we are a part. Our claim is simply this and no more: We cannot endure together as a people without a sufficient level of healthcare for the community as a whole. That claim establishes the moral foundation for a system of universal healthcare, while at the same time limiting our claim for individual cure.

It is striking, moreover, that the progress of the historical first phase—nutrition and sanitation, most decisive for longevity—is far more a reflection of social and living conditions than of medical conditions. It is no less striking that the second historical phase was achieved through (a) concern, not with individual welfare as such, but with the damage done to groups by infectious disease, especially epidemics, and (b) basic biological knowledge, pertinent to human beings in their common features rather than in their particularity. This is not to deny that something similar may one day turn out to be true of many chronic diseases of the third phase; it is just not as likely. One reason for their persistence is that they are multi-factorial in their causality, take many different forms in their expression, and more reflect some fundamental limitations of human biology. The individual variations are numerous and complicated. That makes them amenable neither to simple vaccinations for prevention nor to simple treatments, such as antibiotics, once contracted (though genetic therapy could make a difference here). In that respect, the first and second phases of the medical revolution can be significantly distinguished from the third, current phase.

If our healthcare system (and the social system of which it is a part) did nothing more than keep the conditions of the first two phases in good working order, it would ensure long and healthy lives for the majority of the population. If it only did that, and nothing more, it would be an adequate healthcare system for any nation. If it only did that, and did it well, it would be a reasonably (if not fully) just system, providing a basic benefit for everyone. It would take care of our most important requirements for the exercise of our citizenship and participation in the life of our society. Anything beyond that level would be welcome, but not necessarily required.

Yet that is likely to seem too stringent a standard, not only because a country might be able to afford more, but also because it would leave as a residue some significant problems for particular groups within the population. They fall into two categories. One of them is made up of the health problems that the advances of the first two phases do not fully respond to: accidents, genetically induced illnesses not wholly amenable to behavioral or societal eradication, mental illness, and other conditions that tend to lead to premature though not necessarily early deaths or to a high probability of a life of suffering and disability. The other category is made up of the "third-phase" chronic illnesses and disabilities, especially those that increase in incidence with age, becoming especially pronounced in old age.

What priority should we give these additional categories? That is the real, and economically crucial, question. It is those latter two categories that pose the greatest economic problems, that make most problematic the idea of ultimately conclusive medical progress, and that most bear on uniquely individual well-being. It is the pursuit of success with them that most makes healthcare, as an economic and social category, encroach on other societal domains important to the overall life of communities and societies.

My argument is that, once society has provided the baseline of preventive care and public health I have so far sketched, it has done most of what ought morally to be required of it. With one critical exception—that of providing care (not cure) for each individual in all of his or her individuality—it may consider other health services morally optional and set them aside, if necessary, in the name of other legitimate social goods. But to make that case and to argue for the primacy of caring, I must now move from the bottom up, coming back to the individual.

## THE GOOD OF INDIVIDUALS

I have tried to show the kind of claim we have as citizens on the health resources of society. That claim is one we make in the name of the welfare of the society as a whole. We can reasonably demand, for our common benefit, that there be a healthcare system which provides enough general health to ensure the decent functioning of the society and its main institutions. That was, in fact, the primary rationale behind the universal healthcare systems of most of the European countries, not that of an individual right to healthcare. The benefit is mutual: We all gain, as a society, from each other's good health.

What kind of claim can we, by contrast, make as individuals in all of our individuality? A good society ought to respond to that individuality. It will be a fearful and threatening one if it does not. We will simply be anonymous, replaceable parts. As Larry R. Churchill has nicely put it, "To the extent that we isolate ourselves and count anyone's suffering as insignificant, to that extent is our own humanity diminished."[5] Writ large, our mutual and shared response to the suffering of others is what makes the difference between a merely well-functioning society and a decent and humane one. It is what is conducive to the devising of a rewarding and supportive society, showing us that our existence as identifiable persons, regardless of our economic or societal worth to the collective whole, has a central place. Yet if we cannot guarantee the individual unlimited medical cure of disease, the meeting of all individual curative needs, then what alternative is there to find that central place for the individual? To get at that question, let me see if I can bring to the surface the basic impulse that seems to lie behind our concern for each other in our sickness and disability, and then go beyond that to the provision of healthcare through the government.

To be sick is to be vulnerable. If we are sick enough, we usually look to others for help. We turn to them, they turn to us. Do we, in some sense, owe it to our neighbor to see that he or she has access to healthcare, or should we see it only as an act of charity or benevolence, not strictly required but expressive of our moral feelings? The answer to that question is unclear, for much will depend upon just what is being asked of us. In a general way, however, there is an almost universal sentiment in developed countries that there is some kind of mutual obligation to provide care. What is its basis? It is undoubtedly our shared sense that we cannot, alone or on our own, cope with the ravages of illness and death, even though they are our most private of experiences. We need the help of others, and the provision of healthcare can be understood as an expression of a need for solidarity in our common plight. The important question is not only how we might justify this sense of solidarity, if we assume that justification is needed, but how we choose to articulate it and to encompass it within the social and political systems.

What is it about the sickness of our fellow human beings that most draws our sympathy and desire to be of help? If we can understand that, we have a basis for both the solidarity and for its embodiment in a healthcare system. I believe that it is, above all, the pain and suffering that most disturb us. That is something we can empathize with, sharing as we all do some occasions of pain. We may not know what it is like to suffer a heart attack if we have not had one, but we can understand what it is to feel pain, to experience a desperate shortage of breath, to suffer anxiety and fear. We respond most immediately and directly to that kind of pain and suffering, and it may be the most common and universal impulse behind the drive to help those who are ill. It is more difficult to appreciate so directly the thwarting of other goods and goals that sickness brings to another person—a trip thwarted, a job deferred, for instance. That is not only because we usually have different personal goals, but also because the nature of the deprivation is less instantly palpable to the eye and the imagination than, say, physical pain. In the case of other goods thwarted by illness, moreover, it is possible in many cases for alternatives to be found (even if a lesser choice), or for the deprivation to be adapted to and tolerated. This is rarely so possible with pain and suffering, whose insistence can be powerful, direct, and destructive of any possibilities of secular redemption.

## THE PRIORITY OF CARE OVER CURE

The pain and suffering of individuals should, for all these reasons, always receive a high priority in the healthcare system. They are both essentially private experiences, even though we can often observe their effects. Pain may be defined as a distressing, hurtful sensation in the body. Suffering, by contrast, is a broader, more complex idea. It may be defined, in the case of illness, as a sense of anguish, vulnerability, loss of control, and threat to the integrity of the self.[6] There can be pain without suffering, and suffering without pain. In either case, only I can experience it, and only I can be relieved of it. Of course some degree of pain and suffering can be tolerated, and I do not mean to imply that the relief of *all* pain and suffering would be an appropriate goal for the system. It would not. I am only saying that they are forms of individual need—private, hidden, not directly shareable with others—that most merit our attention and that are most open to our help. It is the vulnerability that illness creates that most requires the response of others. I call that response one of "caring."

The term "caring" has its liabilities. It conveys, for some, sentimentality and softness, a vague ambiance of feeling rather than a systematic effort to make an effective difference. It need not and should not have those connotations. That in itself is symptomatic of the bias toward acute-care, high-technology medicine, with its comfortable presumption that it *does* something for people in contrast to merely holding their hands. Caring might also suggest acting by default; it is then taken to be what we give people if we cannot cure their disease or change their condition, a kind of consolation prize.

That is a biased understanding. Caring can best be understood as a positive emotional and supportive response to the condition and situation of another person, a response whose purpose is to affirm our commitment to their well-being, our willingness to identify with them in their pain and suffering, and our desire to do what we can to relieve their situation. As Dr. Leon Eisenberg has observed about the care provided by physicians, "The comfort that treatment brings—what has been termed 'caring' as opposed to curing—is what accounts for the antiquity and the continuity of the physician's function in society."[7] The caring response can take two related forms. One of them is constituted by the attitudes and personal traits we bring to bear, our concern, sensitivity, dedication, and steadfast patience, for example. The other is the way we socially structure our response: by organizing institutional support when needed, a support oriented toward the provision of comfort and security, assisting the patient to accommodate to his or her situation in some structured way. To care for someone is to give him or her our time, attention, sympathy, and whatever social help we can muster to make the situation bearable and, if not bearable, at least one that never leads to abandonment, the greatest of all medical evils. Caring should always take priority over curing for the most obvious of reasons: There is never any certainty that our illnesses can be cured or our death averted. Eventually they will, and must, triumph. Our victories over sickness and death are always temporary, but our need for support, for caring, in the face of them is always permanent.

Is there not something anachronistic, even archaic, about urging the priority of caring over curing? Does that not undo the very point of scientific medicine, that of finding cures for illness rather than settling for care? Not at all. The steady increase in chronic illness, the almost certain emergence of economic limits on many curative possibilities, and dissatisfaction with impersonal medicine press it once again to the foreground.

The primary assurance we all require is that we will be cared for in our sickness regardless of the likelihood of cure. Of course it is important for the healthcare system as a whole to know how it can prevent disease, and to know what it might do to cure it once individuals are afflicted. But above all it must be prepared to support and minister to people in their vulnerability to sickness and death, which can only be reduced, never vanquished. That is the one assurance we must all have from our fellow citizens and human beings. The greatest failure of contemporary healthcare is that it has tended to overlook this point, has become distracted from it by the glamour of cure and the war against illness and death. At the center of caring should be a commitment never to avert its eyes from, or wash its hands of, someone who is in pain or is suffering, who is disabled or incompetent, who is retarded or demented; that is the most fundamental demand made upon us. It is also the one commitment a healthcare system can almost always make to everyone, the one need that it can reasonably meet. Where the individual need for cure is infinite in its possibilities, the need for caring is much more finite—there is always something we can do for each other.[8] The possibilities of caring are, in that respect, far more self-contained than the possibilities of curing. That is also why their absence is inexcusable.

We might look at caring more closely by attending to the three basic human needs I outlined earlier: the need to exist, the need to think and feel, and the need to function (to act in the world). The threat of death is the most obvious, and extreme, instance of danger to our need to exist. In most people, that threat evokes fear and dread. Even though many seem, in their dying, to be able to accept it, the passage from life to death must stand as the center of the drama of human fate. It is that passage, more than the inconceivable situation of actually being dead, that most grips the imagination, most presses us back upon and into ourselves. As the ultimate form of separation from the human community, those undergoing that passage most need the company and care of others, to keep them socially in the community until the last possible moment, to assure them that they will not be forgotten, that the death of their body will not be preceded by the death of their social self, pushed out of sight and out of mind by fearful medical workers or families. The great value of the hospice movement is its contribution to the care of the dying and to opening up, once again, the possibility of accepting illness and death in an affirmative way.

Consider also our need to think and to feel. In the most extreme cases, those suffering from severe mental illness, dementia, or retardation can seem well beyond caring, so cut off from others that they appear irrevocably trapped within themselves. Care for them can seem useless, yet because there is no clear certainty about what it means to the victim of a severe pathology of mind or emotions, their care becomes important as a way of binding them to the community, a way of treating them with dignity, of recognizing the humanity remaining, however hidden or distorted. For those with lesser conditions, burdened by anxiety, or with distortions of affect, or with mild retardation or dementia, they need the care of others to function in the world, to have it made a safe place for them.

Something similar is true for the handicapped and physically disabled, thwarted in their need to function. They require the assurance that they will not be cut off from the company of those able to move about and act in the world. They will depend upon others to act for them, to move them from place to place if they are in a wheelchair, to read to them if they are blind, to change their underclothes if they cannot do so for themselves, and, most of all, to accept them as still valuable, still cherished members of society. If they are chronically ill, they may suffer some combination of all these needs; for reassurance in the face of death, for help with the emotional stress of a drawn-out, unending illness, for assistance with the physical tasks, the movement, that may gradually come to be beyond them.[9]

I need not elaborate upon the kind of caring that those with different needs will require. It is for the most part well known, and those who work with the afflicted can readily supply the details.[10] At the center of these needs is the experience of illness, disability, and loss of self-control and self-creation that ordinarily accompanies them. Illness is hostile to the integrity of the self, its sense of being at one with and in direction of itself. Sickness alienates us from ourselves first of all, from the familiar, comfortable, healthy body or mind. It sets us at odds with ourselves, and that alienation can quickly spread to a sense of alienation from others, those who remain among the healthy and the active. We feel we will lose the love and respect of others, that if our illness goes on long enough, or is severe enough, it will place us outside the circle of those for whom the world is still comfortably theirs. It is the suffering of illness, not simply the pain it may bring, that most oppresses: our fears about the future, our feeling of loss, our anxiety that control and self-direction are, or may be, no more.

To care for another is to minister to these fears, to supply love and patient fidelity to the anxiety about separation from others. It is to assure another that they remain important to others, that their illness has not deprived them of a life in the community. It is to ease their pain where possible, and then to help them live with their frailty, whether of body, mind, or function. To do this effectively requires skill and insight. The continuing failure of medical education to train students to do this well is revealing. It is surely not because the subject has never been mentioned in discussions of curriculum reform. It has been a perennial topic over the years, but it always loses out to an emphasis on scientific knowledge and technical skills, and there is no end in sight to that bias.[11] Medical education remains overwhelmingly technical in its emphasis, and of course those skills are the most highly rewarded financially. This is hardly to say that doctors are uncaring; most are and only a small proportion are not, at least in my experience. Too often it is nurses who are expected to provide caring, however.

Caring is just not the trait that is emphasized for physicians the way medical knowledge is. The technical skills they deploy are impersonal, directed to organ and system failures, not to the particularities of individual suffering. The ability to care requires a capacity to acknowledge our own mortality and our common vulnerability, as well as to understand the privacy and hiddenness of much pain and suffering in others, an understanding that requires imagination. We are all fellow patients or potential patients, doctors and laypeople alike; that should never be forgotten. The medical educational system has fitfully tried, by rhetoric and exhortation, to bring caring back to the center of medicine. That can hardly work when the enterprise itself is so decisively oriented toward cure, toward aggressive action, toward mastery of the body. That bias pushes, and must push, care to the side. Care will only become central if, and when, medicine shifts its goals and ends.

If the center of caring is the way we respond to another as an individual person, a way of being with that person in all of his or her uniqueness, then its effective manifestation requires institutions, accommodating social structures, and a society prepared to make room for those it cannot cure or return to "productive" life. For the dying, the need may be for that of an institutional hospice, for a solid home-care program, for the kind of psychological and social counseling necessary to ease the passage from life to death—which may be true for the family as well as the dying person. The family may on occasion require legal assistance, and sometimes the help of social workers in trying to hold together in the face of the death of one of its members. For the mentally ill, or retarded, or the elderly demented person, institutional care will be necessary in the most severe cases, and good programs of home care for those not quite so badly off. In still milder cases, counseling of family members may be needed, and vocational help. For the functioning of the disabled, their families will need technical training and psychological counseling to understand how to do what they must do, and how to live with the enormous pressures that being a caretaker can entail. Programs of occupational therapy will be required, as well as a range of community services, most of them going well beyond the narrowly medical.

Again, I need not fill in the details of these familial and institutional needs. However intricate and elaborately structured such institutions may be, the provision of caring of that kind is within the range of finite possibility. A decent, if not perfect, job could be done. I am not claiming that it is inexpensive. It is not. I am also not claiming that it would be possible to do everything that might be imagined in the name of caring. Demand could exceed possibility there as well. I am only claiming that caring does not have about it the inherent infinity of possibilities characteristic of that medicine which aims to cure illness and to forestall death. The individual need for caring is more limited, able to be reasonably well circumscribed in decent social programs and caring individuals.

Where the limitation of curative medicine in the name of the good of the society as a whole—which I believe necessary—courts the danger of an unfeeling utilitarianism, a simultaneous and counterbalancing focus upon individual caring can keep a concern for the individual at the center of the healthcare system. Caring is the foundation stone of respect for human dignity and worth upon which everything else should be built. Its presence can be a steady and faithful one even in the inevitable absence of resources to carry forward the open-ended enterprise of cure. It is in caring that we can address the uniqueness of persons, that which makes them different from each other. It is in caring that we can respect the claims and calls of individuality, that we can most show our solidarity with each other. When all else fails, as it eventually must in the lives of all of us, a society that gives a priority to caring in its response to individuals is worthy of praise.

## ACHIEVING IMPLOSION

By emphasizing the priority of caring over curing in the healthcare system, I have meant, first, to find a goal for the system that meets some fundamental individual needs and yet is at the same time as a general enterprise feasible. That is not true of a goal of the endless cure of disease. I have meant, second, to provide a countervailing, balancing value to the emphasis on societal needs and claims which I have argued should distinguish the enterprise of curative medicine and the kind of scientific progress that has become its characteristic mark. I want to stress, however, that I am speaking the language of "priorities." By that I mean simply to say that some goods and aims should as a rule take precedence over others, that care should generally come before cure as a societal emphasis. A priority does not entail a rigid set of rules, nor does it mean that care must *always* come first. The point of a priority is to give a general bent and coloring to the system. It is not a prescription for inflexibility, and it admits of reasonable exceptions. The enormous suffering, and shortening of life, occasioned by cystic fibrosis in children would, for instance, constitute a reasonable exception. It is a condition that cries out for cure as would some other congenital conditions that manifest themselves in children or young adults.

Yet if we accept the general priority of caring, where and how should space be made or left for the pursuit of curative medicine, by which I mean the effort to eliminate or cure illness, to achieve normal functioning, and to stave off death? The first requirement is that we find a way of bringing the current economic explosion of curative medicine under control, a task that can begin by recognizing that we *already* have a sufficient level of societal health (with some noted exceptions). The second requirement is that we acknowledge the primacy and necessity of providing care for all, and only then pursue our aspiration to move beyond care to cure where sensible and possible.

I approach this complicated task with the image in mind of an implosion. How can we turn the force and intensity of our quest for healthcare inward rather than always outward? A controlled implosion will require two initial features, which will provide the competing forces: a set of limits, and a set of aspirations. Our social task will then be to keep them in appropriate tension, and that task, in turn, will require a set of priorities. I will turn first to the setting of limits.

## Setting Limits: Aging and Individual Need

A system that seeks implosion rather than explosion must, above all, admit of firm limits. That acceptance of limits should build upon some basic, undeniable truths of human existence. The most important of these is that the human body is finite. It is part of its nature to become ill, to age, and eventually to die. At its best—now and forever—medicine can only forestall death and relieve for a time, and only that, the diseases and frailties of the body. An appropriate and prudent goal for medicine is to provide a reasonably healthy life within the framework and limitations of a human life that is, of its nature, finite and bounded. An obsessive pursuit of health, an unwillingness to accept death, and a never-ending struggle against old age are not fitting goals for individuals in their own lives or for a healthcare system.[12]

For all of the good that health represents, there are some important points to keep in mind as it is sought. The most important of these is that *there is no perfect correlation between health and happiness, between length of life and satisfaction with life, or between the health of individuals and their common good as a community*. Good health can help us live better lives, but the final meaning and value of life will not ordinarily turn on the state of our health. More important will be what we make of the living of a life of which health is the means. A recognition of limits can be understood to encompass the acceptance of a full (but not necessarily biologically maximum) life span, death from conditions whose eradication would require an unreasonable expenditure of resources, and a circumscribed place for the pursuit of health as a societal good.

We have now reached that point in medical and health history where an acceptance of limits requires that some important frontiers be restricted, and strong fences with small gates built at those frontiers. This is the only way to make clear to ourselves that we are prepared to live within limits, and it is the only way in practice that we can *ever* hope to manage our healthcare resources in some sensible fashion. There are two frontiers that must be restricted. One of these is along the temporal axis of aging, the other along the curative axis of individual need. The most imperative first step in the institution of restrictions is to acknowledge that both frontiers are open and endless, never to be conquered. They admit of no known natural, self-limiting boundaries, though some have been speculated upon.

*The frontier of aging.* Most of us now alive will die beyond the age of sixty-five. That means that the future of medical progress, at least in terms of dealing with the highest proportion of mortality, lies with the cure or amelioration of conditions afflicting the elderly. There is no dream so powerful for many than that of wholly separating becoming sick and becoming old, of making old age a wholly new, improved state of life, "the beginning of a new life" as one popular slogan has it. That hope is what might be called the modernization of aging. Yet we should know that this is an illusion, even if we can make some substantial progress. No matter what progress is made with the unwanted conditions of old age—sickness, disability, the fading of youthful powers—there will always be others to take their place. The body will insist upon decline and decay, later if not sooner, but always implacably. The cure of one disease or condition will always be followed by another condition requiring cure, and then another, and then another, and so on indefinitely.

While it will no doubt be impossible and undesirable to wholly restrict efforts to extend life at that frontier of aging, we can ask a special question of the societal healthcare system: What is a reasonable length of life to which people can aspire and which we might together seek to attain?[13] I believe that, if we could get most people through a typically full biographical life span, by which I mean the late seventies or early eighties, we will have done them a decent service. By that time most people will have had the opportunity to raise a family, to work, to love, to travel, to enjoy, to make of themselves what they want to be. For many that task will never be completed, and for others it will be completed much sooner. For the system as a whole, however, we can aspire to a common general level, and certainly most people will have done what can be done by their early eighties.

While it is true of course that notions of a decent biographical life span will be different to some extent for different people, it cannot be the obligation of the healthcare system to orient itself to a kind of curative medicine that is hostage to individual life plans and desires beyond a reasonably full life span. That should always be understood as optional on its part. I can understand why someone would want to live to 105, but it is not evident that I am required, as his fellow citizen and fellow human being, to contribute support toward helping him achieve through expensive medical means that highly individualized goal. I should have helped him with preventive medicine early in his life, with immunization as a child, and with decent primary care, but I am not required to help him pursue extended life. We are not required to follow the culture of modernized aging wherever it might lead, especially when we come to know what it will cost, and how little in improved happiness we might get anyway. A society would, then, be well justified in the future to set an age limit on the public provision of expensive, life-extending, curative healthcare (though always required to provide the kind of caring outlined above).

*The frontier of individual cure.* The second limit is on individual cure. If the possibilities of extending life through time are unending (an ever-increasing average life expectancy and a drawing out of old age), so also are the possibilities of effecting the cure of individuals of all ages. Here we encounter the phenomenon of the vertical gap (Chapter 2), which shows that it is increasingly possible to spend ever-larger amounts of money to save the lives of desperately ill individuals (the $1.5 million to $2 million cases). This growing phenomenon makes clear that, however far we go with medical progress for the individual, we can never find a place to tear the cloth that does not leave a ragged edge, that edge which represents the limits of our present knowledge and skills, ever transcendable, never conquerable. That is a frontier we cannot best, and which needs to be restricted also—not necessarily closed altogether, but closed in the sense that we work to erect a strong fence around it, one that has openings for progress, but small, restrictive ones, subject to powerful restraints.

Yet the problem of restricting this frontier is more difficult in principle than restricting the frontier of aging. It is, for one thing, evident that any attempt to do so would be seen, correctly enough, as a challenge to a key feature of our entire way of life—our belief in the unlimited pursuit of progress. It is also, for another, harder to imagine finding a place to draw a line on the provision of curative medicine for individuals than to find a place to draw a line on curative healthcare and life extension for the elderly as a group. In the case of aging at least, there are cultural traditions of what counts as a "full" life, even if the borders are hazy. All efforts to find good individual standards, by contrast, have fared poorly. However well devised, notions of cost-effective care, standards based on "quality of life," or norms of acceptable outcome are not likely to work well for individual cure, particularly if the failure to employ a possible cure would result in a premature death prior to old age. They will run aground on different beliefs of what counts as a benefit, or a decent quality of life, beliefs made problematic precisely because of a constant medical progress able to draw out some benefit, some quality, even in the most severe illnesses.

We must, then, approach this frontier differently than can be possible with aging. Yet we must do so with a willingness, even before we set out, to understand that we must learn to live with restrictions, that one way or another we must abandon the idea of unlimited progress—but not all progress—on the frontier of individual curative need. The question is how to formulate our aspirations—the progress we might pursue—in the context of limits.

## DEVISING ASPIRATIONS

We cannot have, nor should we even try to have, everything that might be conceivable to biomedical research—to be free of all illness, to live to an average age of 100, to have a life utterly devoid of psychological stress, for instance—but we can achieve many of our dreams. The challenge is to devise some that are reasonable, that can be prudently pursued, and that would be conducive to a coherent individual life, one that has aspirations but is willing to understand that, for the good of all, there must be some firm limits. We need to direct future medical progress to goals different than have been common in recent decades and, at the same time, be willing to admit the need for restrictions on heavy expenditures to promote progress.

What might we reasonably aspire to in the pursuit of that medicine (and healthcare) which promises to cure our illnesses and avert our deaths? We know that it is possible to much better understand than we do now the human body, and its ways of thinking and feeling, and to use that knowledge for the cure of illness. We know that basic biomedical research and clever technological application can bring us advances in curing illness and extending life. We know that, for all we know, there is much more that we do not know. Whether endlessly great progress is likely, however, is something we do not know (though it is reasonable to assume), much less what might be its economic costs and its social and cultural consequences. We are coming to know what the frontiers of financial limits impose upon us, but we do not know where the final end of medical progress might be. We have not the faintest idea about that.

What is important for our present societal purposes, however, is to devise a set of *reasonable* aspirations, ones that combine technical feasibility, a thoughtful understanding of what is most conducive to human happiness and welfare, and economic good sense. Scientific possibility and reasonable aspirations are not the same. How can we decide which of the latter to pursue? Let me develop a general way of answering such a question.

It is possible to articulate three reasonable aspirations for biomedical research and its application to curative healthcare. None of them will be readily or quickly realizable, and some may be indefinitely far in the future. Yet it is important to have a sense of direction and some ultimate goals. The goals I propose are imaginable curative goals, within the presently known range of medical possibility (for the most part), and yet at the same time not necessarily open-ended in nature (though some may well turn out to be so). The aspirations for curative medicine are as follows:

1. *The meeting of body needs: a full life span and the avoidance of a premature death.* On the axis of aging the goal would be that of enabling everyone to live out a full biographical (not necessarily biological) life span, by which I mean to the late seventies or early eighties. Efforts to understand, and then cope with, the major causes of premature death would be central to this aspiration, as would be efforts to reduce morbidity within it.

2. *The meeting of cognitive and emotional needs: a psychologically stable mental and emotional state.* To the extent that psychiatric and psychological therapy can assist people in averting or managing the more chronic and pathological conditions—not the ordinary unhappiness and vicissitudes of human existence itself—it should be available and seek to refine its skills, methods, and insights.

3. *The meeting of functional needs: a state of adequate functional capacity.* Rehabilitation, including vocational therapy, should be available to everyone who can profit from it and who can have their capacity to function in the world significantly enhanced.

I state these goals as "aspirations" only. They are ideals toward which we might strive, but ideals which must be put in permanent tension with our acceptance of limits, and particularly (I would hope) the limits on aging and individual need earlier sketched. Each one of the aspirations for cure raises the problem of the vertical gap in trying to meet individual need. We cannot help each and every person to live out a full life span—some medical conditions may be resistant to any curative success, and others would require enormous and disproportionate expenditures. We cannot give everyone psychological stability—some cases will be forever refractory. We could not possibly rehabilitate everyone—some people will remain incapacitated, and it will be difficult to adapt the world to their flourishing. All of this is simply to say that both our aspirations and our sense of limits are real, and that they will be forever in tension, in a struggle, with each other. Our most delicate social and political task is to keep them in fruitful tension.

# CHAPTER 6

# THE DELICATE BALANCE: LIMITS AND ASPIRATIONS

Until very recently, the ethos of healthcare was dominated by lofty aspirations and unbounded hope, by a sense of unlimited opportunity needing only resources, energy, and will. The more sober, to be sure, knew that the agenda of hope was in part unrealistic, but the politics of progress has long required the suppression of sobriety. Dreams and longing command money, not limits and realism. It is the latter we now need. The question before us, then, can be simply stated: How are we to find a decent, workable balance between the limits we should now recognize in all their force and those aspirations that remain valid? That will be an immensely difficult task in practice, even if we can come to some agreement on the conduct of debate, on the boundaries within which we should all work, and on the priorities that, in general, might make the most sense. Our first task, however, is to see if we can settle upon appropriate priorities, ones that would express well the tension most suitable between limits and aspirations. What I want to lay out here is a way of thinking about that problem. Then, in the next chapter, I will address more directly some of the practical problems of implementing it.

The first and most important point to make is that there exists no simple, mechanical formula, either in ethics or in policy, for devising solutions to difficult balancing and priority issues. I have expressed at various points my abiding skepticism of various technical procedures and techniques—cost-benefit analysis and technology assessment, for instance—designed to provide us with clean answers to muddy questions (and will do so some more in the remainder of this chapter). I have constantly used terms such as "reasonable," "sensible," and "prudent"— terms of human art and judgment. I believe these to be the right terms to use, however vague and controverted they are and must remain. But that is the nature of our problem. It requires judgment, not formulas. Our common task is to see if we can invent, and then live by, some common standards for "reasonable" and "sensible," recognizing all the while that they are standards we fashion together out of debate and discussion.

## LIMITS AND ASPIRATIONS: DEVISING POLICY

To make sense of such terms in the context of balancing limits and aspirations we require an allocation policy. By that I mean a broad and organized way of looking at ourselves, our desires, and the limits of the world in which we live and then using it to decide what is, when we cannot have everything, comparatively more or less important. In this instance, we need a policy that gives us a helpful way of looking at the twin demands of limits and aspirations. A "policy" represents a general direction of thought and action, providing a basic framework for making decisions. It is "general" insofar as it does not map out in advance the exact choice to be made in each situation; it allows for contingencies and unforeseen, complicated developments. The policy has a "direction," however, insofar as it tries to affirm and express a given cluster of values and goals; these goals and values will pervade particular choices. As part of its direction, it will specify certain lines—the limits—that should not in the ordinary run of cases be crossed.

I have already signaled a direction for the allocation policy I have in mind—by putting limits before aspirations. That was not a chance ordering. The dominant future policy bias in our system, I contend, should be that of cultivating a sense of boundaries, finding ways of dampening our unbounded hopes and enthusiasms, trying in particular to keep our health aspirations firmly set within a broad perspective on the entire range of individual and social needs. That means having a lively, imaginative awareness of the costs of constant progress, an awareness that becomes as powerful (if not more so) as the present unrestrained capacity to imagine a future of glorious medical triumphs. Fifty years ago, a different policy bias was appropriate. There were many things to be done, and there were growing resources to do them with. Yet it is exactly because we have made such great progress—because our societal health in general is now already so good—that we can afford to shift our bias in a different direction.

Such a bias will make us more fearful of a "successful" cure that we might be unable to prudently pay for than a failure to find the cure at all. Such a bias will make us look first to the risks rather than the benefits, to the pitfalls rather than the opportunities, to the dangers rather than the glories. Such a bias will make us think twice before we indulge our enthusiasms. I well recognize that this is a way of thinking uncongenial to Americans, addicted as we are to the upbeat, to a repudiation of "negative thinking," to a loving caress of dreamy thoughts. But that is the bias now required of us if we are to bring our own system under control and, beyond that, to control the very future of biomedical research and healthcare delivery (in this and every other developed country).

That is an austere recommendation. But is that the end of the matter? No. It is, I stress, a bias only, a direction, not a flat set of rules or inflexible guidelines. Even with such a bias there will be sufficient room for much more medical progress and for improved health and healthcare delivery. Indeed, we will need ongoing research on better ways to provide care, and to improve the quality of life within limits. What I am looking for is a way of cooling down, of dampening, our enthusiasm and hope, not eliminating them. My image is that of the wise and perceptive society, one that still entertains its dreams, but does so now from the perspective of experience and maturity, whose usual lessons are to caution us to take care, to curb imprudent enthusiasms, to watch out for proferred bargains that conceal insupportable costs.

The policy direction for balancing our limits and aspirations I propose we entertain begins, then, with a bias toward limits and restraint. It also needs to contain two particular ingredients. One of these is a perspective on the assessment of technology and on the research imperative. The other ingredient is a strategy for devising priorities, beginning with care for all and then carefully working its way through other health needs, particularly curative needs.

## Assessing Technology, Judging Research

Nothing so characterizes and defines contemporary healthcare as the pursuit of scientific knowledge and technological application. The belief that the key to the cure or amelioration of disease lies in technological progress is deep and abiding, even though there is powerful evidence of long standing that health status is determined by many things other than the availability of state-of-the-art technology. The cost of that progress, in the United States and elsewhere, is enormous. What has been called "intensification of care"—by which is usually meant the application of technological advances and intensified services to individual patient care—accounts for approximately 25 percent of the inflationary cost of healthcare over and above general inflation.[1]

Some of the impact of that intensification can be found in the "vertical gap" I referred to earlier, the great and growing distance between the costs of the least expensive and the most expensive patient. It is the source of the $2 million rescues, and bills that can run into the hundreds of thousands of dollars for a lengthy course of intensive treatment. To be sure, not all of the heavy costs of healthcare can be traced to technological medicine, but even those that cannot will usually display some indirect consequences of technological advance. Thus a person who spends a number of years in a nursing home, at a great cost each year, may well be there because he or she survived an episode of acute illness that would have killed someone in earlier decades, and may remain in the nursing home because routine antibiotics will spare the patient a death that would have come much sooner fifty years ago.

I suggested in Chapter 2 that the present methods of technology assessment cannot be effective unless accompanied by a value framework which can then be employed with it. Those methods can project some costs, some social and other consequences, and develop some future scenarios about their deployment and dissemination. But because their serious application depends, at bottom, on some substantive idea of meeting individual need by which to judge the technology, it is a method that neither can be nor has been effectively and broadly applied to the actual making of difficult decisions. It can work, at best, in those circumstances where a technology is clearly and demonstrably of great value or of no value, or of utterly negligible value; standards of simple efficacy of that kind can be developed. But it does not work effectively where the benefits are marginal (of benefit to some but not all, or of some but not great benefit) or where there is serious disagreement about what counts as a benefit (as there often is with marginal or moderately beneficial technologies).

Is an average life expectancy of five years, in relatively poor health, and at a very high cost, a good or a bad outcome? That is the present situation with kidney dialysis, strenuously defended by its promoters, and that is the expected outcome of the artificial heart, if it is someday finally developed. That heart is expected to provide an average increased individual life expectancy of fifty-four months, including an average of 2.5 additional hospitalizations—at an estimated total cost of $150,000 (1983 dollars).[2] That gain to life expectancy was judged a good enough prospect for the government in 1988 (with some political pressure) to continue a research investment in the artificial heart, now already totaling some $250 million over a period of some twenty years.[3] Since technology assessment, as such, does not in any case provide us with the principles to determine, from an ethical or economic point of view, whether the investment is "worth it" or not, its value is greatly limited. It is a method that can only work if some substantive principles can be brought to bear, from the outside, to allow us to judge the worth of technologies.

What are some principles that might serve that substantive purpose? We might of course say that no technology should be used unless it can carry a 100 percent success rate of cure with good long-term outcomes, but most cannot do that; we might also insist on a 50 percent success rate, but that would be relatively arbitrary. The problem is far worse when we are trying to evaluate the social costs and benefits of technologies that do have a high medical success rate. Technologies that fail, or produce poor medical results, can be forced out or their use restricted; their failures are patent. Those that have good medical results but marginal or uncertain social consequences are more difficult to judge. The hardest technologies morally to judge— and to determine whether to reject—are those that are both medically and socially successful and expensive to use. They are the ones in the long run that drive up the cost of the system, the ones that keep forever luring us from one ragged edge to another. We need principles that can point us in prudent directions, and I advance two such principles. I will call them the principles of symmetry, and of technology assessment.

## The Principle of Health Symmetry

The principle of symmetry is this: A technology should be judged by its likelihood of enhancing a good balance between the extension and saving of life and the quality of life. Its aim is to promote medical coherence, by which I mean outcomes that foster the rounded well-being of persons, not simply one-dimensional improvements that benefit some aspect of individual well-being at the expense of others. No technology can guarantee a rounded outcome in this sense, but if well developed it can promise a high probability of such a result. That should be the aim in devising it and a standard of judgment in disseminating and financially supporting it.

A healthcare system that develops and institutionalizes a life-saving technology which has the common result of leaving people chronically ill or with a poor quality of life ignores the principle of symmetry. The saving of very low-birthweight babies at the cost of a poor long-term outcome is an example, as is that of using cardiopulmonary resuscitation (CPR) in those cases where the resulting quality of life is likely to be poor. More generally, entitlement programs (such as Medicare) that reward and reimburse well the use of high-technology procedures, but do not well support caring for the lasting damage perhaps done by them or that do not provide long-term care as generously as high-technology care, also by analogy violate the principle of symmetry.

The principle would require the pursuit of research promising an acceptable and balanced *long-term* outcome, not simply an immediate benefit. This would mean giving priority to the development of technologies that promote long-term benefits, that seek a good balance between life extension and quality of life, and that seek also to minimize the impact of illness on those already afflicted. Here are some possible specifications, couched in terms of goals to be pursued:

*Pursuing those avenues of medical research that promise a good long-term, overall outcome (at the lowest general cost, financial and otherwise).* Research priorities should be given to those conditions where the state of scientific knowledge and the likelihood of successful clinical application and outcome are the highest over the longest period of time. This principle would imply a bias toward relief of those conditions which are relatively well understood, which predominantly affect children and younger adults, and which promise to enhance the likelihood of avoiding a premature death. Beyond that general priority, the goal should be to pursue research possibilities with the most beneficial long-term results. While this would seem an obvious point, the eager pursuit of such devices as the artificial heart (mainly of value to middle-age males and promising, even if successful, a relatively short enhanced life span of four to five years) indicates that it is in practice far from accepted.

*Pursuing those forms of healthcare that strike a good balance between the saving of life and the maintenance of a good quality of life.* A powerful proclivity toward acute-care, high-technology medicine has been the mark of the past fifty years or so. This bias has meant the neglect of those conditions that do not shorten life but significantly reduce its quality: arthritis and incontinence among the elderly, as well as poor long-term and home care; inadequate rehabilitation services and financing for the victims of accidents; and genetic anomalies among younger age groups. A primary question always to be asked is: If we are to have available life-saving therapies and technologies, do we also have in place other follow-up therapies and forms of care that help ensure a good long-term quality of life? If the answer to that question is no, then there should be a strong reluctance to disseminate the therapy until such a standard can reasonably be assured. Therapies that promote a good quality of life—hip replacement in the elderly, speech therapy in children—even if they do not extend life, should be given priority in such cases.

*Pursuing those forms of healthcare and research that provide the best help for those already born with defects and handicaps; working to reduce the impact of illnesses already incurred.* Medicine overreaches itself when it sets as its implicit goal that of curing all diseases and indefinitely forestalling death. Since one consequence, moreover, of an unrestrained effort to hold off death by technological innovation is often that of producing chronic illness and disability in its wake, medical progress of that kind assures the production of still more illness. That cycle can only be broken by developing technology to meet the needs of those who have already survived and whose lives promise long suffering, whether physical or psychological. We should also give priority to those who can be saved by existing technologies over the saving of still more lives by the creation of still more new technologies designed to press beyond present frontiers. We should not, in short, go beyond those frontiers until we know how to improve life for those already existing, but poorly, within the present frontiers. To use a military analogy: If we are going to conduct a war on various diseases, we should not extend our advance beyond our supply lines. That is the classic way of turning victory into defeat.

## Principles of Technology Assessment

How are we to judge the success or failure of a technology? I advance the following principle. A technology should be judged a failure, or a distinct societal threat, under two circumstances: when it medically fails to achieve, or achieve well, its stated purpose; and when its success would tend to create significant distortions in the healthcare system, especially that of threatening societally necessary limits on the frontiers of aging and individual need. There are, then, problems of failure and problems of success.

The problems of failure are well known and are the almost exclusive focus of current efforts at technology assessment. The generally accepted standard of failure would be something like this: Is an existing technology, or a proposed new technology, one that would be efficacious in its use? If it is not, or would not be, efficacious (or only marginally so) then its use may be curtailed or eliminated (by refusal, say, of government reimbursement of its use). How rigorous the standard of efficacy ought to be will depend upon our willingness to tolerate discretion and choice in the use of a technology, and how stringent we believe our budgetary constraints to be. In vitro fertilization to relieve infertility has a success rate of less than 20 percent after repeated, and expensive, attempts. Yet some states have mandated insurance coverage for what is, by any standard (save that of hope and desire), a relatively inefficacious technology. The great difficulty in judging whether a technology is efficacious is too often the lack of any consensus on what constitutes waste or inefficiency, and on the nature of patient benefit.[4] But of course it is precisely to make such determinations that technology assessment is wanted in the first place; thus the exercise itself has a deep flaw at its very heart. Even so, unfortunately, the necessity of determining when a technology is wasteful, or insufficiently beneficial to patients, remains.

However important for immediate cost-containment purposes, technologies that fail, or produce marginal results only, do not pose the most serious economic or moral problems. They can justifiably be eliminated. That is not true of effective technologies, those that bring real benefit. It is what works, and undeniably so—but at a high individual or aggregate economic cost—that poses the hardest moral dilemmas for the development of an affordable system of care. An artificial heart that fails can be eliminated. But one that would save thousands of lives, and provide those it saved with some additional years of life, would be a great additional financial burden on the system, and all the more painful to deal with because of its success and of the demand that success would generate. A highly expensive drug that would extend the lives of victims of AIDS for a number of years, such as AZT, would be another example, as would the use of total parenteral nutrition (TPN), now growing, for the same group of patients. We need, then, to have a way of thinking about the possible impact of relatively efficacious, but expensive, technological developments. I suggest, therefore, the principle of technological success: A technology that might achieve a short-term medical success but may generate long-term medical or social problems requires special scrutiny and considerable resistance. The purpose of this principle is to force us to ask questions that might otherwise be avoided. What we need, and do not have, is an art of assessing the implications of medical success. I simply offer the kinds of questions that present an agenda for the development of that art; in the meantime, they are questions that should give us pause as we consider particular forms of technological progress.

*Weighing the medical consequences of success.* Too often the only test of a new technology is whether it brings immediate relief to a medical problem. But what are its likely long-term medical consequences?[5] If it is a therapy that will cure a disease or save a life, what will be the state of the life that has been saved and the societal implications of saving such lives? We need also now to ask of a proposed technology what it will mean for the overall life of the patient, not simply the immediate good of the body. Will a new diagnostic procedure effectively replace older ones, or will it simply provide a marginal gain on already available technologies, with only a small medical gain in general patient welfare? If the diagnostic gain will be a major one, do services exist to provide the therapeutic benefits necessary to take advantage of the diagnosis? If so, what will be the medical consequences of those benefits?

*Weighing the societal implications of success.* We now know that the saving of life, the providing of rehabilitation, and the cure of illness can have social implications. It changes the fate of individuals and their relationship with others, makes a difference in the welfare and dynamic of family life, and can alter the social structure of society. The combined success of effective contraception (leading to smaller families) and the extension of life spans (leading to more elderly) changes the ratio of young to old, with great social consequences. The "success" of acute-care medicine, for example, has increased the burden of chronic illness, both on society and on families. Thousands of head-injury victims are now being saved who would have died even a few decades ago (a 400 percent increase in recent years in the number of teenage head-injury victims); they require long and arduous care in many instances. Over a long enough period of time the aggregate impact of changes of that kind and magnitude begins to fashion a different kind of society. How should we think about those implications? What kind of a society do we want, and what kind of medicine is most conducive to it? What kind of medicine do we want, knowing that different kinds of medicine are likely to lead to different kinds of society over the long run?

*Weighing the cultural impact of success.* It is the success of medicine that encourages us to want still more of it. Our expectations are raised. We flirt with ideas of invulnerability. We imagine our old age as one of new excitement and wonderful changes, not of decline like our parents, or their parents. Medicine and good healthcare come to symbolize a triumph over the forces of finitude and entropy. Medical breakthroughs excite the public because they bring hope, hope that the world is not fated to go against us, that it can in some sense be transcended. But how much and what kinds of expectations of that sort, of that stimulation of hope, are good for us? At what point are we led to forget our inherent limitations? When do we begin resting too much hope on medical progress to bring a transcendence of the failing and limited body, or of the depressed spirit? At what point does the success of medicine lure us, as we allocate resources, to investing more in it to meet our present needs than to take account of the likely needs of future generations? At what point do the possibilities for extending the life of the elderly, with this new medical procedure or that, distract our attention from the educational, or welfare, needs of children—of modernizing one stage of life, the last, at the possible expense of those who have yet even to live a full life? At what point does the possibility of technologically improving the outcome of neonatal care for low-birthweight infants turn our eyes from the desperate need of some frail elderly people for decent home care? What does that, in turn, do to our cultural values and ideals of our relative duties to young and old?

In suggesting some directions for future technology assessment, I mean in particular to stress the necessity of first identifying, and then debating, the moral, societal, and cultural ends we want the technology to serve, and then trying to judge the technologies in light of those ends. What has instead been sought with technology assessment as now practiced is some kind of neutral technique, one that could be used to serve any end that society agreed upon or that represented some political consensus. But it should now be obvious that the assessment process itself must encompass a reflection upon goals and ends and itself contribute to articulating and shaping them. Otherwise, technology assessment cannot be carried out effectively, nor can its result be of any meaningful kind. A mode of technology assessment that knew it had to judge technologies by the symmetry they promised to promote, by the need to stay within limits, and by the necessity of taking into account long-term societal goods could have a center and a gravity now lacking, and necessarily lacking.

## Judging the research imperative

A long-standing and powerful belief in the value of scientific research is a fundamental part of the American healthcare system.[6] That belief responds to the general commitment to science and technology that is part of our culture, and to the specific faith in its efficacy that has long been part of the modern biomedical crusade. Two issues concerning that faith are of importance for my analysis. Will the investment of more research money eventually bring down the costs of care? Is it worth directing research funds to what James F. Fries has called the "compression of morbidity," that is, reducing the length and intensity of illness prior to death in old age? Let me first put those two questions in context.

*Will an investment in research generate eventual healthcare savings?* It is possible to imagine a direct challenge to the approach I am proposing. That would be to embrace my proposed goals—to agree, for instance, on the value of limits, the principle of symmetry, and the dangers of thoughtless success—and yet say that a still greater investment in basic biomedical research and technological application would be the best way to get there. It is of course perfectly *conceivable* that future research could discover exceedingly inexpensive ways of treating the most costly and difficult problems on the frontiers of aging and of individual need.[7] One argument of this kind relies on the possibility that we will discover inexpensive ways of dealing with the basic causes of costly illnesses—a preventive vaccine to replace expensive therapies is a common model to embody this kind of hope. Another argument is that, as expensive technologies are refined, their cost can be brought down to acceptable levels; further research investment toward that end is therefore justified.

These are not arguments to be dismissed out of hand. They have some plausibility based on historical experience. But their force is less than potent, requiring not outright rejection but a response that is measured and wary, putting a heavy burden of proof on those who deploy them. The fact that inexpensive cures were found for many diseases in the past does not guarantee they will be discovered for all diseases in the future, especially for the present array of chronic diseases. The fact that some technologies become significantly less expensive over time does not mean that all future ones will. Nor does that view take account of the fact that the cheaper a technology the more extensive its use will be, and that a medical system made up of a large number of relatively inexpensive technologies taken individually can add up to a large total bill. The straight-line correlation, documented by the National Institutes of Health, between an investment in research and healthcare costs indicates a very low probability that that will actually happen. The correlation evident in Figure 2 of the appendix (p. 276) suggests the folly of depending upon more research to reduce costs substantially.

Those who propose further research investments in the name of meeting as-yet-unmet individual needs, or as a way of bringing greater efficiency and cost containment, should be asked some probing questions, of a kind embodying the standards for the assessment of technology suggested above: (1) If the research or technology development should be a success, what are likely to be the medical, societal, and cultural consequences, and are they desirable and affordable? (2) If success at the present ragged edge of meeting individual need could be attained, what would be the next ragged edge it would in turn expose, and what would then be the problems of coping with that edge? (3) Will the improved technology promote symmetry, that is, a good balance between length of life and quality of life, for instance? (4) Would the same amount of money invested in some other societal need be as likely, or more likely, to improve the overall state of society? Finally, what would count as good answers to questions of that kind? Good answers, I contend, would make use of reasonably hard, reasonably solid evidence, not hope and aspiration.

*Investing in the compression of morbidity.* James F. Fries of the Stanford University Medical School has been untiring in his advocacy of a shift of research priorities away from expensive life-extending technological medicine to preventive medicine and the "compression of morbidity." It is a powerful and important idea, and one wholly consistent with the way I have been trying to morally and socially analyze the provision of healthcare. Its most potent attraction is that it offers a scientific rationale for a major shift in research and technology priorities, one that could reduce costs in the long run as well as produce improved health. Its very attractiveness—the promise of symmetry it offers—is precisely why a certain caution is necessary in assessing its plausibility. It seems all too nicely, as a theory, to solve many of our most pressing problems; the world does not often turn out that way.

Fries begins with the commonly held belief that the life span of the human species is finite, fixed by our genetic nature. Our goal, a feasible one, should be to postpone the time at which we become victims (as we inevitably will) of some chronic disease which will eventually kill us. The later the onset of that disease, the more we have compressed morbidity, and with that compression thereby reduced the individual and social burden of illness. An important healthcare consequence of the theory, if true, is that it "puts emphasis on prevention rather than cure, postponement rather than palliation, and personal autonomy [management of personal health-related behavior] rather than paternalistic care."[8] The main evidence Fries offers in support of this theory (and attendant healthcare strategy) is evidence in favor of the finitude of the human life span, and a "rectangularizing" of "survival curves" (later illness, but not later death). A number of recent studies, he contends, show that health-promotion and disease-prevention programs bring about just such a result, that of people who are healthy and active later and later in life without necessarily having a longer individual life span.

I will not try here to examine in detail the evidence he offers. It is interesting and suggestive, even if it has its vigorous critics.[9] I earlier argued that, since death always wins in the end, it would be naive to think that we can banish the high costs of healthcare simply by curing disease; the elimination of death by one disease in a person just sets the stage for death by another. Fries agrees that "elimination of a particular illness from a particular life does not automatically mean that that life will contain less morbidity."[10] Something even more severe may take its place. But not necessarily or inevitably. On the whole, he believes, the exchange, or trade-off, can be a positive one in many cases, with the result a final illness less costly and less extended than might otherwise have been the case. Working with his premises, the major healthcare goal should be that of research efforts to postpone the onset of chronic illness and systematic efforts at disease prevention, using available present knowledge to achieve that postponement.

We do not, it seems to me, have to fully accept the hypothesized scientific basis of the "compression of morbidity" theory to make prudent use of its healthcare strategy. We can, through research and health-promotion efforts, work to reduce atherosclerosis, cancer, emphysema, osteoarthritis, and memory and hearing loss (to take a few examples), knowing at the least that we are improving the symmetry of the system, enhancing quality of life without investing money in further extending life by means of high technology. This will be particularly valuable in healthcare for the elderly, but will benefit other groups as well. It would move us toward giving a low priority to what might increase general life expectancy, but a high priority to that which will relieve the onset and burden of chronic illness, now the main source of illness and death. It would, as Dr. Alexander Leaf, Professor of Preventive Medicine at the Harvard Medical School, has emphasized, lead to a healthcare system that tried to "keep people as . . . healthy, vigorous, and productive as long as their biological life span will permit." Dr. Leaf also notes, "We are spending more money to buy the wrong thing, namely to keep people alive as long as possible rather than buying health."[11]

## Setting General Healthcare Priorities

I have laid out a somewhat complex scheme in the preceding pages and it may be helpful to bring it together in a summary form. In a previous chapter I tried to outline a way of determining the relative priority that should be given to healthcare, proposing that we already have enough good health on average in this country but that, in any case, in the principles of sufficiency and full accounting we could have a strategy for coming to some societal determination on that issue. I also claimed that a society is fully justified in looking primarily (not exclusively) to societal rather than to individual benefit in the provision of curative healthcare—that which saves and extends lives. In Chapter 5, I then developed the case that a countervailing emphasis on the provision of care for all—given the inherent impossibility of cure for all—would offset the utilitarian flavor of a system based on societal welfare and represent a feasible possibility. At the same time, I began developing a strategy for setting priorities in the pursuit of a cure for disease and a forestalling of death. Those priorities are, first of all, to be set within a context of limits—limits to an extension of old age and to the pursuit of individual cure—and then, from there on, to be subject to varying tests and questions.

Imagine a pyramid. At the base, we provide care for all, then move on to the provision of those ingredients of public health that enhance the health opportunities of all. We do all we can not to stint at that level—it brings the greatest general benefits. After that, the pyramid begins to narrow, and becomes all the narrower in allowing possibilities for expensive technological cures—that is, those cures directed at individual illnesses, of a kind that fall through the net of general public health measures and initiatives. Eventually, we will have spent all the money we can afford, and our restrictions on further expenditures, our actual limit-setting, will come as we approach the top of the pyramid, as we move into the area of high-technology, expensive individual cure or averting of death.

The various levels of care can be categorized as follows:

LEVEL 1: The provision of caring in its most basic forms: the (topical) relief of pain; hospice or comparable care for the dying; nursing or home care and companionship for the elderly and otherwise frail; simple mental health programs for the mildly disturbed; basic and decent home and institutional care for the chronically ill, the demented, the disabled, the retarded, the severely mentally ill—all those powerless to care for themselves

It is Level 1 that sets the basic moral agenda and its baseline of healthcare. It is not only important in its own right; it also should pervade all the other levels.

LEVEL 2: The provision of nutrition, sanitation, a tolerably clean environment, and programs of occupational health, preventive medicine, and health promotion, including accident prevention and prenatal care

LEVEL 3: The provision of immunization and protection against infectious disease, and antibiotics and antimicrobials to control infection

LEVEL 4: The provision of emergency medicine and primary care, but limited to routine, relatively inexpensive forms of diagnosis and therapy (e.g., immediate life-saving and emergency-care, palliation of pain, and simple forms of surgery and rehabilitation)

The provision of healthcare through the first four levels addresses (on the whole) those threats to personal integrity and health that are shared by almost everyone in a society, regardless of individual differences. Money invested at these levels will produce the greatest impact on mortality and morbidity, and will do so at the lowest cost per capita.[12] Money invested in caring ensures the preservation of human dignity in the face of illness, the greatest individual need. Levels 5 and 6 below, by contrast, come increasingly to address individualized problems, a threat to some (perhaps many) but not a common threat to all. There will be no precise line between these two general categories, and scientific knowledge will affect the way we categorize the nature of the threat to societal or individual health. Yet they are sufficiently solid that they could effectively be used for policy purposes.[13]

LEVEL 5: General, advanced forms of medical cure or restoration (e.g., advanced surgery, cancer chemotherapy, extensive rehabilitation)

LEVEL 6: The provision of highly advanced, technological medical therapy (e.g., dialysis, open-heart surgery, organ transplants, total parenteral nutrition)

In devising a healthcare system, Levels 1 through 4 take priority. The provision of care at these levels makes the greatest contribution to the common good, not only because the largest number of people can be helped at the lowest cost there, but also because if those four levels of care can be provided the result will be a level of health and dignity sufficient to ensure adequate functioning of societal institutions, formal and informal. The foundational place given to caring means that the public-interest focus of Levels 2, 3, and 4 is decisively softened and humanized by a core place for individual need; it provides the point of departure. It is only at Levels 5 and 6 that severe limitations on individual needs—individual curative needs—begin to make their appearance.

Before turning to the problem of dealing with those limitations, a further question is necessary about the various levels. Would it not make sense to increase the research investment so that the conditions of Levels 5 and 6 could eventually be dealt with less expensively at the lower levels? Not necessarily. That has by no means been the invariable outcome of earlier research and, in any event, the chronic diseases that are now dominant do not seem as likely to be as amenable to such an approach, and certainly not at a low research cost. In listening to pleas for more research funds on the promised ground of eventually reducing healthcare costs, we should remind ourselves again and again of the message shown in Figure 2 of the appendix: Healthcare costs may and probably will go up in any case, and probably precisely because of the possibilities for cure research can turn up. A research agenda designed to lower long-term healthcare costs is not, I emphasize, a goal to be dismissed out of hand. It is an idea worth pursuing with energy, but it is no less an idea that requires a powerful memory of past failures—recent history is not bunk here—and a sharp, appraising ear when such promise is hyperbolically bandied about, as will surely happen in future congressional hearings on research budgets. It is most likely true that there are great future scientific advances possible. It is most likely not true that the pursuit of those advances is a valid long-term strategy to reduce healthcare costs.

## SETTING CURATIVE PRIORITIES

Before suggesting an approach to setting curative priorities, a caution is in order. The temptation to believe that, with enough ingenuity, a quantitative or other specific calculus to set priorities might be possible is powerful. It appeals to our love of tidiness and our belief in efficiency; a parade of numbers, somehow, carries in our culture a weight of authority that the verbal and qualitative do not. "Numbers," a prominent policy analyst was reported to have said, "bypass values." That is a grand illusion. In a world of comparisons, of disparate human goods and ills, of different personal responses and meaning—a world of hip replacements and neonatal care and psychotherapy and liver transplants and physical rehabilitation—quantification of relative values will not be possible. These comparisons will, for policy and allocation purposes, have to be left to the political process, which cannot guarantee truth or final goodness, but only—at its best—a sense of a fair procedure and a chance for values and proposals to clash in some illuminating and acceptable way. If numbers cannot be the final answer, and no precise calculus will be possible, what can be done? We can decide what questions we want to ask as part of the political struggle, and we can determine some general policy bias or inclination within which to situate the struggle.

The policy bias I propose is, first, that with Levels 1 through 4 the burden of proof for *not* providing such healthcare lies with the government and its elected representatives. Since healthcare through those four levels so patently serves justice and the public interest—the general good of society and the effective functioning of its critical institutions—it would be derelict to scant them unless some compelling reasons can be offered to do so. No such reasons exist in our society. With levels 5 and 6, however, there should be a shift in the burden of proof. Since at that point the benefits focus more on disparate and varied individual needs, the burden should be relatively more upon individuals to show that a claim for cure should be societally honored in the face of medical scarcity and other societal needs. The societal obligation is lessened because it cannot responsibly be discharged. The "burden of proof," however, need not be a fixed burden. In times of affluence and expanding productivity and national wealth, it might be relatively easy to discharge. In tighter, more straightened times, it would be more difficult to discharge. At present—with a powerful need to control costs, and with a high level of average health, a decent sufficiency—it should be used to establish high, demanding standards. The burden of proof should be heavy.

How might this work in practice? We would need a set of

standards against which to measure various claims for curative medicine. We would not, with such standards, have a precise instrument to determine the burden of proof, but we would have enough key ingredients for a sensible public debate. We would know what we ought to be arguing about and what we ought to be comparing. I will provide a possible list of such standards, compatible with the principles and perspectives earlier advanced:

## Standards for Priority Evaluation of Curative Medicine

1. Promise of serving public interest by:

   a. Meeting special age-group needs (e.g., physical mobility for mothers of young children)

   b. Meeting special socioeconomic needs—"principle of balance" (e.g., prenatal care for low-income women)

   c. Reducing infectious potential (e.g., programs to reduce sexually transmitted disease, especially AIDS)

2. Promise of relieving long-term care demand by:

   a. Promoting independence in daily living (e.g., relief of severe arthritis)

   b. Relieving or reducing institutional burden (e.g., drug regimen making possible deinstitutionalization)

   c. Relieving or reducing familial burdens (e.g., cure or amelioration of Alzheimer's disease)

3. Promise of meeting basic human needs:

   a. Body needs:

      i. Basic life-saving survival need (e.g., liver transplant)

      ii. Relief of potential risk to life (e.g., cure of hypertension)

**b.** Psychological needs:

    **i.** Relief of seriously crippling mental illness (e.g., schizophrenia or deep depression)

    **ii.** Relief of milder mental illness or emotional disturbance (e.g., phobias)

**c.** Function needs:

    **i.** Restoration of basic function necessary for daily living (e.g., sight, hearing, speech, mobility)

    **ii.** Restoration of bodily function *not* necessary for daily living but important part of normal human potential (e.g., relief of infertility, athletic disability)

**4.** Efficacy and acceptability of curative treatment:

    **a.** Efficacy of treatment (e.g., high, moderate, low?)

    **b.** Satisfies "symmetry principle"—that is, good balance between length and quality of life (e.g., well, moderately, poorly?)

    **c.** Long-term medical, social, and cultural consequences (e.g., good, moderate, poor?)

    **d.** Good cost-benefit or cost-effective ratio—using best available economic techniques (e.g., high, moderate, low?)

How would a list of this kind be used? It would simply serve as a systematic checklist of pertinent criteria to be used in evaluating a particular form of curative medicine. It is a list of those points that ought to be considered, and a list that goes well beyond immediate medical benefits. At the end of such an exercise a legislator or policymaker would have achieved a good overall appraisal, one integrating a number of different perspectives. That would then provide the basis for a meaningful political debate (which would encompass the relative priority to be accorded the various categories on the list), a debate that would ordinarily take place in a context that might impose a severe, or relatively light, burden of proof on individuals seeking help. Similar sets of standards would be needed for the evaluation of proposed diagnostic procedures and technologies, and for research priorities, but I will not try to develop them here.

There is one thing missing from this list that might seem essential—a set of priorities for using the standards themselves. I would suggest two general priorities only, that a heavy weight be given to long-term benefits, and to meeting special age-group and socioeconomic needs. The great need is to put in place a healthcare system that can stand the test of time, and not generate new crises every few years. With those exceptions, no clear priorities need to be set. But are not some of the standards more important than others—is the meeting of a life-threatening body need inherently more important a consideration than, say, efficacy of treatment, or a body need more important than a function need? Not necessarily. A universal set of decisive priorities cannot readily or adequately be developed to answer questions of that kind. We will differ among ourselves (and sometimes with ourselves) and much will, in any event, depend upon circumstances. If a body need for survival can be met only using a very expensive treatment of poor efficacy, that would not necessarily take precedence over relief of neurotic psychological problems using inexpensive methods of proven high efficacy. That is just the kind of issue, however, that we should leave to the political process.

Making use of that process, it is quite possible and feasible that a particular community—a city, a state, a program—could work out an acceptable set of priorities, one that commanded general assent. I am only saying it does not seem feasible to develop a *universal* set of priorities, to be used in any and all circumstances. The important requirement is that the political process have solid standards and criteria with which to work; that is the purpose of the lists. It is possible that, after rigorous debate, priorities would begin sorting themselves out. The initial policy bias would, of course, make a great difference, and that is why determining what it should be would be the first step in a policy debate. In our present circumstance, that bias should be to place a heavy burden of proof on those who would support expensive technologies devoted to individual cure. We have more pressing societal needs in general, and more pressing medical needs in particular.

# CHAPTER 7

# DEVISING A POLITICAL STRATEGY: CAN WE GET THERE FROM HERE?

The American healthcare system will and must change. Sheer necessity—the economic and organizational strains of the present, increasingly unworkable, system—is forcing it to do so. Reform proposals are common, but usually piecemeal in their character, focusing primarily on financing mechanisms rather than the cultural contexts and values that have generated so many of the present problems. It is hard to discern in them a coherent picture of a viable future system. The reason for that void may not be hard to understand. Most reformers have wanted to work within the present set of national values about health, hoping that by devising some ingenious fresh mix of them, a new system could be born. But those values, for all of their attractiveness taken one by one, are when taken together hostile to a coherent, just, and economically plausible system.

We will have to change not just the mix and balance of the values, but the values themselves. What are they? They are those of autonomy and free choice, of a commitment to unlimited medical progress, of a belief in always-improved quality, of a rejection of the effects of aging, and of an ambitious dedication to the eradication of all pain and suffering. To that general list, we must add the specific values of different interest groups, each seeking to maximize its own welfare. There are the economic interest groups: physicians and healthcare workers, the manufacturers of drugs and equipment, the administrators of hospitals and healthcare systems. There are the health interest groups: the various disease-oriented societies (the American Cancer Society, or groups concerned with AIDS, or Alzheimer's disease, or leukemia, for instance) as well as the interest groups that press for the health welfare of different age groups, whether children or the elderly. There are the research interest groups: those seeking money, for example, for basic biological research (usually in the name of some eventual health benefit).

While we might in the case of each of these interest groups debate who is or is not getting a fair share, not one of them represents an illegitimate interest or concern. They are expressive of deep and abiding values—jobs, profits, the conquest of disease, and scientific research. Our political system, moreover, blesses the legitimacy of interest groups, allowing them to seek their own good in a singleminded way. It is someone else's task to figure out how to balance and blend the interests. All of this amounts to a system that, taken as a whole, is neither an organized system nor a coherent pattern of activities. Many of those values will have to be changed or modified as well. They generate a collection of needs, demands, practices, and customs that work against each other and that promise, if left unrestricted, to subvert any serious reform efforts.

In the short run, there are two pressing social requirements, apparently incompatible; taken together, they bring us to the center of the healthcare problem. One of these is the need to provide a more equitable, and full, base of healthcare support, particularly for the poor and near-poor, and then for those middle-class working people threatened with the economic devastation of a major illness. It is hard to imagine how that can be achieved inexpensively. The other requirement is to find a way to control the ever-rising costs of healthcare, especially the cost of expensive entitlement programs, particularly Medicaid and Medicare, and of private insurance plans. It is hard to imagine how that can be achieved without reducing expenses and cutting back on healthcare. Our deepest immediate societal needs, therefore, work in contradictory directions.

Those short-run needs are symptomatic of still deeper issues, and they constitute our long-run requirements. The matter of equitable healthcare presses us to consider more fully the place of health in society and the extent of resources that should be devoted to it, just as it presses us to ask what counts as just and fair in attempting to meet individual needs, needs that we now know are limitless if they are for the curing of disease. The issue of controlling costs compels us to think about the relationship between health and human happiness, and the economic implications of that relationship; about learning to live with the gap between what we might like and what we can learn to tolerate; and about the way we are politically to balance individual need and societal possibility. Taken together these long-term problems also force us to consider an appropriate balance between two different possible goals of a healthcare system: one that aims to provide maximum equality and one that aims to provide maximum health.[1]

In the previous chapters I proposed a set of approaches—and ultimately a different set of values—to meet these problems. I now want to see just what it might take, politically, to make them feasible. My perspective is ultimately long term. The changes I believe necessary would probably take a generation or more to accomplish, but now is the time to begin that process.

## GOALS OF THE HEALTHCARE SYSTEM

There can be no significant, long-lasting reform of the healthcare system unless there is a reasonably coherent set of goals that commands a significant national consensus. I offer here an articulation of goals I think plausible, based on the analysis of the preceding chapters:

*The primary goal of the healthcare system should be to provide those general measures of public health and basic medical care most likely to benefit the common health of the population as a whole, and to ensure that every person in the society receives care, comfort, and support in the face of illness, aging, decline, and death.*

*The secondary goal of the system should be—within the limits of a reasonable level of healthcare expenditures in relationship to other societal needs—to pursue a basic understanding of the causes of illness and death, and to aspire to the cure of those illnesses that bring premature death and thwart common human aspirations.*

*The emphasis of the primary goal falls upon societal health needs and the common individual need for caring in the face of sickness. The emphasis of the secondary goal falls on the pursuit of the cure of those forms of illness most likely to express individual differences and to thwart individual need.*

Flesh can be put upon the bones of my proposed goals by thinking of the healthcare system as composed of three levels, at each of which change will be necessary. The first level is that of our way of life, that is, the way we bring our deepest moral and political values to bear on the fashioning of a healthcare system. I will call this the *cultural level,* where we embody the values of our way of life. What do we take to be the relationship between health and human happiness? How important is it to attempt to relieve human suffering, to ward off diseases, to resist aging, decline, and death? It is at this level that our way of looking at and understanding ourselves and the world most comes to bear. It is the level that, explicitly or implicitly, is most likely to shape everything else we do. It provides us with our most basic premises and predilections, our deepest rational and emotional commitments. For any serious change to take place, it is the most important place to begin—even though it may be the hardest to change. It was the purpose of my earlier chapters to bring this level to the center of our attention.

The second level bears on our notions of a right or entitlement to healthcare, and our beliefs about who has an obligation to provide or ensure good healthcare and how it is to be financed. Here we begin to confront different ideas about what a just healthcare system should be, as well as various notions about the kinds of duties we owe to each other as individuals, both sick and well. In one sense, questions of societal justice and fairness come to the fore here; in another sense, questions of individual rights and obligations are no less important. I will call this the *entitlement level*.

The third level encompasses all of the institutions, mechanisms, and modalities by which healthcare is actually provided to people: the hospitals and clinics; the acute and long-term care facilities; inpatient and outpatient care; the work of physicians, nurses, and other healthcare workers; and so on. It is through these institutions and mechanisms that we embody and implement our values about health and our notions of justice, rights, and obligations. It can be called the *institutional level*.

Any significant changes in the way we think about, and provide, healthcare need to work with all three levels, and more or less simultaneously, most importantly beginning with the first. A failure to do this accounts for the collapse of many recent reform efforts. The cost-containment movement has so far failed because it has been unwilling to confront directly, much less to challenge, the deep philosophical and cultural values, principles, and ways of life that underlie the institutional mechanisms of the present system. It has tried to manipulate the system at the institutional level within the context of accepted values; that effort cannot succeed. Various efforts to determine what would count as a just and equitable system of healthcare rights and entitlements have, in their turn, no less failed to confront the way of life that underlies the system and to face up to the practical difficulties of achieving equity without enormous changes in institutional mechanisms. However difficult it will be to work with all three levels at the same time, only an effort of that kind is likely to be sufficient for the task at hand, nothing less than a fresh direction for the healthcare system of the future.

## SPECIFIC GOALS FOR THE THREE LEVELS _____

How can the general structure of the healthcare system suggested above be given a new configuration at each of the three levels? I propose the following ideas as principal ingredients:

1. *Health and Ways of Life—The Cultural Level*
   —Good health is to be pursued in order to enhance individual flourishing and societal welfare
   —Health is a means to human well-being, not an end in itself; good health does not ensure happiness, and happiness does not require perfect health
   —Aging, sickness, decline, and death are part of the human condition; an unlimited pursuit of health to escape those conditions is a distortion of sensible human ends and purposes
   —A wise society will set limits to its aspirations and expenditures for life extension on the frontier of aging and on the frontier of the individual cure of disease
   —A society has a sufficient level of health when its citizens are on the whole healthy enough to pursue its common purposes and participate in the life of its private communities, and when poor health is in general no longer an impediment to the functioning of its major social and political institutions

2. *Justice and the Healthcare System—The Entitlement Level*
   —Since it is impossible ultimately to defeat death, a just and sensible system is one that tries to strike a balance between caring and curing, with primacy given to caring, the most fundamental human need; those in pain, the chronically ill, the retarded, the demented, the handicapped, and the dying have priority
   —An equitable and rational healthcare system is one that provides a guaranteed minimal level of adequate care for all; it is, at the same time, one that is prepared to set upper limits to the pursuit of im-

proved individual health if that is necessary to achieve the guaranteed minimal level

—A "minimal level of adequate care" consists, first, of full support for caring (that assistance, and those institutions, that sick, dying, and disabled individuals need to tolerably bear the burdens of their condition); second, of full support of those public health measures that promote general societal health as well as access to primary and emergency care; and, third, of access to more individualized forms of cure compatible with a sensible allocation of resources to the health sector in relationship to other societal requirements

—A just healthcare system is compatible with three levels of access: one that guarantees a minimal level of care and cure for all, a second that allows individuals and their employers to mutually agree upon benefit packages, and a third that allows the use of personal income for the pursuit of health beyond either of the first two levels

3. *Organization and Efficiency—The Institutional Level*
—Individual choice pertinent to caring should be as broad and individualized as is economically feasible

—While choice is a valuable human good, an efficient and just healthcare system is not always compatible with full freedom of individual choice, particularly for the pursuit of cure, on the part of either patients or healthcare providers

—Limitations on freedom of choice should be based on broad, participatory discussion, established by appropriate and visible public or institutional authority, subject to change based on experience, and guided by equitable rules and procedures; it must be assumed that not everyone will be satisfied with the results

—Medical technologies should not be publicly or

professionally sanctioned unless they can be shown to be significantly efficacious in achieving their intended goals, cost effective in their dissemination, and beneficial in their long-term medical, social, and cultural consequences

—Research priorities should be directed to improving the quality of life of those already burdened with illness or disability rather than determining how to further extend life; to those conditions and circumstances most likely to produce long-term benefits; and to prevention strategies and the compression of morbidity

—A rational healthcare system requires a significant degree of central planning and management, and this will be especially important in organizing a system that guarantees a minimal level of adequate care for all on a national level

—No entitlement program for curative medicine should be established that does not set limits on its benefits, and it should be prepared, if necessary for effectiveness, to set those limits by using categorical standards rather than by relying on individual patient or physician discretion

The ingredients I have proposed for a coherent, fair, and economically manageable system raise a large number of practical moral and political problems, and they must be considered. Before doing so, however, it is necessary to clarify the relationship between the public and the private spheres in healthcare.

## PUBLIC AND PRIVATE ROLES

By talking in general about the "healthcare system" I have left vague the relationship between the public and private sectors. That was deliberate. The first question we need to consider is the nature of health, then what we want the organized forces of society to contribute to the maintenance of our health, and only then take up the question of just who should carry out that task. That issue is now at hand in my analysis, and I begin with a simple assertion, increasingly less controversial: Both the complexity and the expense of modern healthcare require a central government role even if considerable room can be made for the private sector. Biomedical research, on the one hand, and the delivery of healthcare, on the other, require a concentration of resources and organizational skills appropriate to state action. I have suggested that, in thinking about healthcare, we could best classify it with defense, fire, and police protection, that is, as a general societal need. Even though we have different individual needs and demands, illness represents a common threat and defense against it should be seen as a common, shared enterprise.

The actual history of healthcare in America has, however, been very different. With the exception of some early public health activities, it was not until well into the twentieth century that government began to play a strong role in the health arena, by the establishment of the National Institutes of Health in the late 1930s, by the Hill-Burton Act in support of hospital construction in 1946, and by the initiation of the Medicare and Medicaid programs in 1965. The domination of fee-for-service medicine, centering on the individual patient paying the individual doctor for his or her services, symbolized the early belief that healthcare should, for the most part, be left to the private sector. It was the very success of medicine in curing disease and extending life, and the recognition that its implications and organization transcended private agreements and relationships, that brought government in, and guarantees that government will remain there. At the same time, the early history and traditions of American medicine linger on. They embody a strong and continuing suspicion of government, the relative neglect of public health, and a powerful role for the private sector as a source of services and as an occasion for considerable profit.

Much of the incoherence of the present system can be traced to the awkward marriage of the public and private spheres. It is a marriage of convenience, for each has come to need and depend upon the other. It is no less a marriage of a couple with different interests, values, and histories. The future of the healthcare system depends upon how this marriage develops. One point is evident: the stronger the public demand for health-care, the more valuable what healthcare has to offer, the more confused and inequitable the actual access to and payment for that care, then the greater the role of government will, and must, become.

The fact that every other developed country (save for South Africa) has given a major role to government coordination and financing of healthcare, and has provided a foundation for universal care, reflects not simply a greater willingness elsewhere to turn to government, though that is true enough. It also reflects a faster realization that modern healthcare systems are too complex and interdependent to be left to the vagaries of the market; the market cannot efficiently and effectively do what is necessary. As Robert G. Evans, the eminent Canadian economist, has observed, "Universal coverage is a necessary condition for government to engage in bilateral negotiations, to exercise the leverage whereby cost escalation can be controlled."[2] The United States, resistant to the end, is now being forced to go in the same direction. That is because, as others earlier discovered, there is no other viable alternative, at least if there is to be any sustained drive to meet health needs in a reasonably efficient way. No more than we can afford to organize private armies and fire brigades can we any longer depend upon private medicine and private financing to take care of us adequately.

What is a feasible and appropriate role for government? To answer this question we might look not just to theory, but to the actual roles that have emerged in recent decades and to the forces that have driven them. The most fundamental role has been, first, that of leadership in organizing basic biomedical research, an expensive and complicated enterprise and one where the usual financial rewards required of private corporate research efforts cannot always be assured. Only government can afford a costly research enterprise that does not have to financially prove itself with immediate benefits. A second role has been that of enforcing various public health measures and of filling in the gaps in the delivery of healthcare, attempting to meet the needs of those unable to afford healthcare through the market system (or in the workplace). Just as there are many kinds of basic research that will not return a profit to the private sector, there are many categories of sick people whose care will not do so either. Government stepped in because a failure to have done so would have led to unacceptable deprivations—of the fruits of basic research knowledge, on the one hand, and of available healthcare benefits for large numbers of people, on the other. The third basic role has been that of regulating standards of research and practice, licensing healthcare professionals, and carrying out various oversight functions.

That basic rationale for a strong government role remains valid. It is a crucial focal point for goading and channeling the research enterprise, for meeting public health needs, and for promoting a fair allocation of health resources. An acceptance of the analogy between healthcare delivery and other protections of the common good (defense, fire, police protection) would further strengthen that role and lead to a greater emphasis upon those forms of research and delivery benefitting the populace in general rather than just individuals. As a general rule, the place of government in the healthcare system should be that of promoting the public interest, leaving to the private sector the meeting of the special curative needs and demands of individuals. No sharp line can, of course, be drawn here—there will be overlap and unclear borders. Government must retain some powerful interest in individual well-being just as the private sector should be expected to show decent concern for the public good. But as a matter of emphasis, it is the public good that is the appropriate focus of government action.

A number of specific roles for government are appropriate in that respect:

1. Leadership in, and provision of support for, basic biomedical research and for research on modes and effectiveness of healthcare delivery

2. Collection and analysis of health data and data on the effectiveness of modes of healthcare delivery.

3. Organization of an effective system of technology assessment and dissemination of its results

4. Organization and promotion of public health measures, including programs of disease prevention and health promotion

5. Taking the lead, in its entitlement and public health programs, in establishing coherent sets of limits on the provision of healthcare (including, by means of strict policies on reimbursements for allowable procedures and therapies, efforts to dampen private initiatives likely to skew the overall system or create unacceptable demands upon the public sector)

6. Creation and management of a system of national health insurance designed to guarantee a minimal level of adequate healthcare for all, and to do so in a way consistent with a priority given to caring and to the provision of those services most likely to maximize general health (whether this should be an entirely federal program, or a combined state-federal one, is less important than that there be a program, and a strong one)

The priority of government in its interest in curative medicine, I have argued, should be that of the health of society as a whole, with an emphasis on caring in its approach to the individual. Can that priority be made consistent with a goal of equity for curing as well as caring? That is important, for it would be unacceptable to have a system that, while egalitarian in its concern for caring, allowed egregious disparities in its allocation of resources for curing. At the same time, as I have tried to show, the meeting of all individual curative needs is impossible, and any effort to achieve full equality at that level will and must fail; that kind of effort will do harm to the common good. Is there a way out of that dilemma?

I suggest that, in the form of what I will call the *principle of balance,* there is. In devising health policy, we should see groups of individuals as the basic social units for purposes of allocating curative resources, not individuals as such. The ultimate goal of a principle of balance would be to make every effort to assure that no major social group in the society was, as a group, significantly deprived of benefits available to the population as a whole. The focus of entitlement policy would be on disadvantaged groups, and within that focus an emphasis would appropriately be placed on attending to those general, rather than individual, circumstances that do harm to the group as a whole. Prenatal care for poor women is, for instance, a more sensible priority to reduce the number and damage of low-birthweight babies than the expansion of neonatal medicine to cope with babies born under harmful circumstances; meeting the group needs of poor women would be a justifiable priority even if this meant curtailing services for those individual babies. Priorities of this kind can, of course, be achieved only by systemwide planning and resource allocation.

While there are a number of possibilities for determining what might be the most relevant groups for such balancing purposes, those of age and socioeconomic status seem the most promising. They are familiar and readily identifiable categories. We can, with age, think in terms of the life cycle as a whole (childhood, young adulthood, the middle years, and old age) and ask just what it is that people most need at different stages in their lives. That provides us with the possibility of determining both reasonable aspirations and prudent limits (and we will have to incorporate issues of intergenerational fairness and balance in here as well; children, for instance, should have some priority over adults, and particularly priority over the elderly). Age also correlates well (though not perfectly) with health status, with of course a rising curve of illness with aging. Socioeconomic status also correlates well with health status, for it is as clear as anything can be that poverty and poor health are closely associated. An emphasis on balance would, then, aim to see that no age group was significantly deprived relative to benefits given other age groups (as now happens between the old and the young) and that no socioeconomic group was substantially disadvantaged relative to other groups (though a poor individual might well be deprived relative to a rich one; but the aim here is group, not individual equality—and then not perfect equality, but serious efforts to reduce glaring differences). Inequalities are most likely to be accepted if the most disadvantaged have a decently high baseline of healthcare. If their own health prospects are good, they will be more likely to tolerate the fact that the prospects of others are marginally superior.

A principal task of government would be to devise public programs aimed at reducing age-group and socioeconomic gaps and applying pressure in the private sector designed to stimulate a similar concern. Government can also play an important role in determining, and then helping to do something about, the relationship between those social conditions and circumstances that indirectly produce poor health (poverty, ignorance, and poor housing, for instance). A good society should be understood as one that seeks, then, to achieve a good balance among the significant social groups in the society in meeting their health needs. Every individual as individual has a deep and full claim on care; and every individual, as a member of an age and socioeconomic group, has a claim that the group of which he or she is a part will achieve a balanced proportion of those healthcare resources devoted to the cure of illness.

## DILEMMAS OF IMPLEMENTATION

While there will be no shortage of pertinent considerations for judging the combination of ingredients for a healthcare system of the kind that I have laid out, four in particular are of special importance: the relationship between centralized health planning and individual market choices; the relative role of government and private financing of healthcare; the legitimacy of group or categorical standards for limit-setting rather than individualized decisions; and the moral rights and obligations of doctors, patients, administrators, and legislators.

## Central Planning and Private Choice

There is no secret about the ability of other developed nations to manage costs much better than the United States. The strong, centralized hand of government is the thread that binds together their efforts, even if many of the details of their systems differ. Though they are now also beginning to experience the strains of the triple dynamic of aging, technological progress, and public demand, they are in a far stronger position to cope with them than is the United States at present. Planning, they have long known, is essential to meld the different parts of the system into an orchestrated whole (e.g., closely integrating acute and long-term care for the elderly), thus helping to provide a coordinated range of services for patients as well as enhancing the chance that efficiencies in one part of the system will not be offset by wasteful practices in another.[3] Central regulation can help assure relatively fair and evenhanded treatment through the national system, the control of the introduction and continued use of expensive technologies, and equitable management of costly resources and services.[4] Neither planning nor regulation will, however, be effective without careful oversight and monitoring of policies and procedures.

What do I mean by central planning? I would envision Congress giving the Health Care Financing Administration (HCFA)—or a newly created agency—in coordination with other federal health agencies, the authority to establish national standards on a minimal guaranteed level of care for individuals, on limits to entitlement programs, and on standards for reimbursement for the use of technologies. It would also have authority to mandate specific public health and other programs aimed at the societal good as well as to set standards for physician fees under entitlement programs. This central planning effort should work closely with the states, allowing many details to be left in their hands (but only in ways consistent with general guidelines). The general point would be to invest HCFA with the necessary authority to guarantee access to care at a minimal level and to control those elements of the healthcare system that generate high costs.

## The Relative Role of Government and Private Financing of Healthcare

If there is ever to be a full and comprehensive program of providing a minimally adequate and guaranteed level of healthcare, the federal government will almost certainly have to provide it and, to a significant degree, guide it. Will there, however, be a way to overcome the resistance such a policy will encounter? A three-tier system offers that possibility.[5] It would let government play the major role, at the first tier, as the financing agent and as organizer and coordinator of programs designed to provide a decent minimum level of care for the poor. There appears no way any other arrangement could achieve that end (though the government role is compatible with working through private insurers, and need not be a directly government-run program). At the second tier, the majority of Americans could receive healthcare as part of employee benefit programs, with perhaps a government role to assist small businesses and to promote some uniform minimal standard for corporate programs. At the third tier, the market could be allowed to flourish, allowing people to buy out of their own pocket that additional care not provided by government or by private employers.

This is in principle not too different from the system we now have in a crude form. But it is necessary to make it more openly legitimate, to work to improve its many failings, and to make it humane enough to overcome the animus of many egalitarians against anything other than one-tier medicine.[6] It is also necessary to make it more formal, to make certain that there is, in the end, a comprehensive overall system that does not allow anyone to fall through the cracks.

There would surely be problems with a three-tier arrangement. If there was not some overall effort to dampen general healthcare desires and aspirations—which would necessitate public debate about the place of health in our individual lives and in our way of life—then the first two tiers would be under constant, unrelenting pressure to provide improved coverage. That would most likely provoke a sense of outrage among some. People would be forced to buy out of their own pockets benefits that they would see not as discretionary consumer items, but as critical to their life and well-being. These would not be easy, or pleasant, problems to manage, but they seem preferable to our present ones, which generate comparable chaos and heartache and still offer no good long-term solution.

The most obvious obstacle to a strong government role in providing a baseline of care is that it will require additional, and considerable, government expenditures. This seems inescapable, and the problem that will have to be faced by the American people and their legislators is a relatively stark and clear one. Either there will be a guaranteed minimum level of healthcare for all, and some protection for middle-income people as well, or it is certain that there will be nasty, capricious, and inhumane shortages and discriminations in the future healthcare system, far worse than anything already known. For almost a decade now, there has been strong resistance to an increase in general taxes, and that has been the main reason why talk of national health insurance began to fade in the late 1970s (combined of course with the perception that healthcare costs could not readily be controlled under existing entitlement programs, much less new ones). Can that be changed? I am not certain. Resistance to significantly higher taxes seems strong.[7] It will be imperative to convince the public that a continuation of the present system will do them great and growing harm. They must see higher taxes as a lesser evil.[8]

Of course, a way of averting a direct confrontation over taxes is that of placing most of the burden for a minimal level of care upon business, itself a form of taxation, but one more hidden than a general tax increase. The drawback of plans of that kind so far offered is that they would not provide coverage for all poor people even under the best of circumstances, probably could cost much more than their promoters now project, and place upon business a burden that makes no special sense. Why should businesses have to bear the brunt of a problem they did not create and which, when closely examined, reflects problems in society as a whole, not in the business community?[9] If the business community wants to avoid this burden, then it should take the lead in pressing for an increase in taxes for all. If it is unwilling to do so, then there is a good chance it will be seen as an easier sacrificial victim for the high costs than any other group with available assets. It would be far preferable to prod, and assist, business in making its role in the second tier a strong one, leaving the most difficult financial burden of care for the indigent to government and its general revenue.

## Making Decisions—Categorical or Individual?

When we have to set limits, or establish treatment standards, is that best done on an individual, case-by-case basis, or by the use of what I will call categorical standards? In general, I believe, it will become increasingly necessary to move a long way toward categorical standards and to firm protocols for treatment. The most common norm at present is that of individual physician judgment, usually but not always in consultation with patients and their families. These judgments are ordinarily based on loose, often tacit professional standards and practices, and often as well on the personal standards of physicians. The work of John Wennberg and others, in examining great variations among surgical operations for the same condition in different geographical regions, has decisively established that these judgments can vary enormously, with no visible basis in actual evaluation of efficacy.[10] By a categorical standard I mean, in contrast, the use of some relatively objective, required public standard for the provision of particular forms of healthcare, or for the cessation or limiting of care. Examples would be the use of age as a limit on some forms of treatment for the elderly (and

the main way of restricting that frontier), and the use of firm
outcome or other efficacy standards for other patients (as the
main way of restricting the frontier of individual curative need).
The effort of Lee Goldman and his colleagues to devise a computer protocol to determine whether patients with chest pains
should be admitted to a coronary care unit is suggestive of one
important initiative in this respect.[11] Such standards may be that
of, say, a minimal weight limit for premature newborns as a
condition for aggressive efforts to preserve the life of the baby (as
in Sweden); firm, objective criteria for admission to intensive
care units (as is now the case in many American hospitals, but
implemented in too loose a fashion); the relative likelihood of
significant benefit based on some objective standard from a
treatment (in order that it will be reimbursed); or the elimination
of some expensive forms of therapy altogether, whatever their
benefit, on grounds of cost or relatively poor long-term outcomes.

The attraction of individual decisions by individual
physicians—will this patient benefit from this treatment?—is
that they seem most to respect our differences as persons, both
in what we want and in our physical condition. They are, in that
respect, consistent with the individualism of our culture and
with the moral traditions of medicine, oriented as they are to
individual patient welfare and considerable physician discretion. They are among our most cherished values.

How can I possibly argue that such deep and revered standards may have to be set aside or modified in many circumstances? There are three reasons. The first is that, in the face of
the limitless possibilities of cure, it will utterly be out of the
question for a society to do everything that might benefit individual patients. The demand for maximum individual choice
and benefit is itself a powerful source of our problem. Is there an
alternative? Yes. If a limit must be set, it will be much less of an
assault upon individual dignity to deny a patient curative, beneficial care because of a limit set upon an entire group with a
uniform standard than because it is *this* patient. It would be, that
is, the relative efficacy of a treatment, or its availability to a

particular group—based upon publicly announced and openly visible standards—that would determine treatment reimbursement, not subjective physician, patient, or family judgments about treatment efficacy, or about relative patient worth or quality of life. Individuals can be brought to understand and accept that society might not be able to give them all they want or need. But that will be possible only if it is done in a way that shows they are not being singled out for special discrimination because of who they are personally, and only if they believe that the general good of society is thereby being served. They must, of course, always have the assurance that, if they cannot have all the curative medicine they might want, they will never be abandoned. They will always receive basic care for the relief of pain and suffering—categorical limits would be used only to set limits to curative medicine, not to the provision of care and caring.

The second reason is that, as it is turning out, it is simply impossible to carry out large-scale rationing and limitation policies at the bedside. We know from well over two decades of trying how hard it is to make termination decisions with individual patients even when the desire is simply to serve the welfare of the patient without resource allocation being a consideration. Physicians differ among themselves, family members disagree, and sometimes doctors and patients cannot agree. The important moral tradition that always gives the benefit of doubt to treatment, and the no less potent tradition of medical ethics which does exactly the same, together work to make it exceedingly difficult to stop treatment or deny any possibly beneficial procedures or tests, so much so that overtreatment or unwanted treatment may be common. If asked, then, to carry out rationing policies at the bedside, those traditions would not only put physicians in the unsavory and painful position of having to personally execute policies of limits and rationing with their individual patients, but there is also every likelihood that it would not work in any case. It would invite both evasion of general standards and the application of personal, perhaps capricious, standards, unfair and insensitive in many cases.

Categorical standards, imposed from the outside and setting limits to the actions of physicians in a decisive way, would avoid those problems.[12] The goal would be not so much to tell physicians in oppressive detail what they must do in treating patients as it would be to establish standards of what would not be acceptable at the outer boundaries. It would be imperative that physicians have a central role in helping to set such standards. They must be compatible with physician integrity, and that integrity need not entail a claim that every patient has a maximum claim on maximum resources whatever the societal costs.

The third reason is that categorical standards are open to inspection, are subject to debate, and are clean and clear in their application. That is why they have proved attractive in many other public policy contexts, where an individualized approach would not work well: the setting of a minimal age to drive, to drink, to vote, or to serve in the armed forces; the use of a specific speed limit on highways; and the use of hard standards on vision and hearing for, say, airline pilots and drivers. Inevitably, categorical standards are unfair to individuals; we are different as individuals. But the overall balance of fairness and policy clarity can make categorical standards valuable for public programs. We would, with a three-tier system, allow discretion with those forms of care paid for by individuals. But if it is a government program, one designed to serve primarily the public interest rather than attempt to meet individual curative need, then categorical standards have much to commend them. They would not be perfect, but they could be reasonable. HMOs and managed-care systems would no less be justified in employing categorical standards (though this could be softened by the degree of choice provided people in selecting among different healthcare plans).

There are, to be sure, different ways categorical standards could be employed—firmly or softly. A firm way would simply be to set, for example, the age of eighty as the cutoff point for Medicare entitlements for expensive forms of high-technology care—and to make no exceptions. A softer way might simply be to say that, beyond eighty, a number of criteria would have to be applied before reimbursement would be possible (e.g., a functional assessment indicating that a patient would, if operated upon, have a strong probability of surviving for another five years in good condition). In the case of coronary bypass surgery, to choose another example, reimbursement would occur if stringent conditions for that procedure were met. In a case of expensive rehabilitation, only certainty of benefit based on experience of good outcome with certain categories of treatment would justify treatment. In setting standards—whether they will be firm or soft—much will depend upon how stringent the limits must be, a function of available resources. The softer the standards, the more likely that they will not work well or that they will be abused, even if they promote greater sensitivity to individual variation, which of course they would. The firmer the standards, the more effective they would be as boundaries. One way or the other, however, categorical standards are likely to be the key to any successful setting of limits. No other serious option is available. All others will certainly continue to fail in the future as they have in the past.[13]

## Who Should Decide—Doctors, Patients, Administrators, or Legislators?

The economic viability of any future healthcare system will depend upon its ability to control progress and costs on the frontiers of curative medicine—indeed, to be able to resist those frontiers. But there is unlikely to be an economic success in such an effort without a correlative political success. Both the public and professionals must accept that kind of control and be willing to endure the scarcities and denials it would entail. How can the possibilities for that kind of political acceptance be enhanced? The public must first come to understand the impossibility, the genuine folly, of pursuing individual cure on the frontier of progress whatever the cost and social implications. As part of that understanding, it must no less learn to be exceedingly skeptical of claims that the progress will eventually save money, a claim certain to be advanced. The public should understand as well the feasibility of providing a comprehensive system of care combined with a system of cure that can provide a decent level of general societal health. The public must, in short, be presented with some viable and coherent options to the present system and be able to debate their comparative merits. A vital condition for this to be even possible is that the public must have a chance to take part in sustained discussions of the issues and must be made central to any effort to devise a decent healthcare system. Any final decision-making process should incorporate a meaningful place for all those who have a stake in the outcome, most notably doctors, patients, administrators, and legislators.

I will offer a snapshot portrait of what that participation might look like under my approach to the issues. The most crucial and wide-ranging decisions—the setting of general societal priorities for the place of healthcare among all social needs and for the comparative place of curing and caring in the healthcare system—should be understood as political. Those decisions should be taken at the legislative level, preceded and accompanied by public forums, hearings, and education programs. The system of grass-roots discussion and debate for the general public pioneered in the Oregon Health Decisions program provides an excellent model of how this can work (and the experience of the Louis Harris survey cited earlier in changing public opinion indicates its potential effectiveness).[14] In Oregon and elsewhere citizen groups in local communities have taken part in probing public discussions and debates on healthcare issues, and then have met in larger plenary sessions to compare ideas and exchange insights. It has been a valuable experience for the participants and useful to legislators as well. The task of the legislature will be to put in place a comprehensive government role in the provision of healthcare, distinguishing carefully in the process its role and the role of the private sector. Where categorical standards are required to set limits and establish program and reimbursement standards, legislatures should devise the general criteria, but leave to administrators the actual details (as is now commonly the case with federal programs).

Administrators will have the job of implementing legislative mandates and managing healthcare systems and institutions. Theirs will be the task of seeing that legislative directives are faithfully and fairly carried out in a way sensitive to the needs of those affected by them. One federal agency, either the Health Care Financing Administration or a newly formed agency, should have central national planning and implementation authority, buttressed by a strong congressional mandate and closely integrated with state activities.

What should be the role of physicians in such a system? Or, to put the matter differently: Should doctors make rationing and limiting decisions at the bedside? The common answer to that question is no, and that seems the right answer.[15] Physicians should have a strong voice in the shaping of legislation and general standards, along with the public. Once set, those standards should guide their behavior and set limits to their practice; that will necessarily restrict their professional judgment and discretion to some extent. Yet they should, within those limits, be free to work out with their patients the most appropriate and feasible mode of treatment. To leave the entire decision in their hands—whether and how to ration care—saddles them with what is a societal problem and, in any event, invites an intolerable variety of private standards. To leave the entire decision in the hands of administrators courts rigid and insensitive standards. The compromise solution is for administrators to set the general norms and limits and then to leave physicians quite free to use their best judgments within those boundaries. Regular and formal means and occasions for interaction between physicians in implementing policies would allow for adjustments based on experience. This has been the characteristic method of organizing responsibility in other developed nations, and there is no reason it could not work in the United States. Where it will fall to physicians to implement policies of treatment limitation, they should be fully protected from the threat of lawsuits or legal harassment. It should be understood that they are only working within the guidelines legally established and given them.[16]

For a system of this kind to have any possibility of working, however, it will be necessary to change not only physician behavior but some ideals and aspirations as well.[17] Physicians who feel constantly thwarted in their desire to do what they consider best for their patients, and patients who come to feel that they are constantly being given less than optimal care, will not be just personally unhappy. They are likely also to subvert the larger political decisions that have shaped the situations of which they are a part. That likelihood emphasizes all the more the necessity to bring about a broad public and professional change in the view of health and way of life that underlies the drive for ever-improved curative medicine; and then to have common and sustained discussion on the standards to be binding upon all.

Though I believe they know it well enough in their bones, the training, incentives, and systems of healthcare delivery of which physicians are a part stimulate a view of individual patient welfare that places far too high a premium on aggressive, technological curative medicine. Thus individual patient welfare has become tantamount to providing a particular kind of healthcare, narrowly defined and narrowly provided. We need not only to change societal goals, but also to move away from a one-dimensional conception of patient well-being. The capacity of the present system to stimulate unlimited hopes, to lead to demands for optimal cure, and to engender resentment when desires are not met or procedures cost too much to afford is extraordinary. The most important task is to change characteristic attitudes and expectations, to curb public desire and want, and to bring about a better understanding of the relationship between health and happiness. If there is no success with that task, both patients and their physicians will feel frustrated and angry. As matters now stand, physicians are already increasingly unhappy. They are having standards and practices imposed upon them without their consultative contribution, and nothing whatever is being done to stimulate the more basic examination of underlying values, which I have tried to show is critical for real change. New bureaucratic tyrannies are being imposed on old values, an intolerable combination.

What is it reasonable to expect of patients—which we will all at some time be—as we think about our own welfare and needs, and as we relate them to the larger necessities of the society as a whole? It is unreasonable of us any longer to expect medicine to seek a cure for every disease that might bring us down or to find a method of rehabilitating us in the face of all injuries or the burdens of chronic illness. It is unreasonable for us as patients to forget the needs of society as a whole, or the needs of socio-economic groups other than our own, or the needs of those suffering from other illnesses.

Perhaps the deepest moral pain of severe illness is that it turns us back into ourselves, absorbing all of our energies and sopping up for its own relief the feelings and generosities we would normally reserve for the needs of others. It is that passion for survival or the regaining of our bodily or mental integrity that drives us to seek a cure. Yet that passion, understandable enough in our own lives, cannot be the only or final basis for establishing national or regional policy, or seeking the common good. To that challenge must be brought the more demanding passion of altruism, of a social vision that does justice to a wide range of needs, and of an understanding of health—dug deeply into our consciousness—that recognizes the lack of perfect identity between health and happiness. That is a formidable task for public education, but it is exactly the task before us.

Our behavior must be changed as well, in order that we can if at all possible avoid becoming sick. It is reasonable to expect people to take care of their own health, to live in a way that minimizes their chances of becoming ill. Health promotion as general policy, and pressures on individuals to behave in ways good for their health, should be high future priorities.[18] A distinction is necessary here, however, between positive efforts to promote good health behavior and negative sanctions to punish a failure to do so. While positive efforts are not ordinarily seen as controversial, they easily could become so, particularly if health "education" or "promotion" takes on a manipulative or coercive flavor.[19] Whether people should be directly punished for a failure to take care of themselves (to give up smoking, for instance)—by denial of care, by crippling insurance surcharges or a denial of insurance altogether—is an issue less clear than many would make it.[20]

There should be no special problem with offering incentives for those who live healthy lives, but both the practical problems of enforcing punitive standards (we can tell whether someone smokes, but it is harder to control diet and exercise patterns) and the genuine difficulties of understanding the hidden dynamism of individual behavior make that a method to be approached warily. A doctor can and should work with a patient to see an unhealthy pattern of behavior changed, but it would offend the ethic of medicine—which has traditionally treated sinners and saints—for the doctor to refuse to treat a patient who refused to reform or failed in efforts to do so. It is impossible for physicians to determine ultimate culpability, even for those actions that appear subject to free choice. A system based on penalties for unhealthy behavior would run a severe risk of injustice. Better to use standards that apply to all in allocating resources, the virtuous and reckless alike. The fact that bad health behavior brings its own punishment is (with education programs to point that out) itself a good incentive for individual change. We do not want a system that rewards poor health behavior and sickness. Neither do we want one that treats the ill as willful reprobates, even if some in fact are just that.

It is, finally, reasonable for us as patients to ask our neighbor as a taxpayer to care for us if we cannot care for ourselves. We cannot ask that neighbor for an ultimate cure of disease, or to relieve us of the burden of having bodies that age and die; and we cannot ask the medical profession or the political order for that kind of benefit either. We can ask that our illnesses and disabilities, our threat of death, be acknowledged and the burden of coping with them be shared by others. We can as patients ask of our doctors that they bring their skills to bear on us, that they be our undivided advocates. But we can also ask that, when they act as citizens and as members of professional associations, they consider the needs of patients in the context of other societal needs and priorities. We should want them to speak on our behalf as patients, or patients-to-be, but we should never allow that advocacy to make greater claims for the importance of health, or the economic priority of medicine, than good sense and wisdom allow. Just what that "good sense and wisdom" should be must be the subject of an ongoing dialogue among patients, physicians, and government.

One additional way to understand the political task before us is to think of it as an effort to change the way we understand "quality" and the way we should politically and economically pursue it. If we continue to define high-quality healthcare as requiring the constant improvement of that care, the use of the latest and the best in technology, and always-enhanced outcomes, then the chase for quality is an endless one and the chances of achieving any lasting efficiency are rendered impossible. If doctors and patients work with this image of "quality" in mind, they will never be satisfied and will never learn to live within some prudent limits (or will do so only by virtue of gross coercion).

Quality care should be understood as the best form of care possible with available resources, that form of care that represents a good balance between individual needs and societal possibilities. Increasingly, it should be understood that quality is possible within a steady-state healthcare system, one that seeks to achieve a decent level of care and to remain there. It is both unnecessary and often harmful to use as a standard of quality constant improvement. If "quality" is forever joined with the idea of progress as its necessary twin, then we will frustrate ourselves in seeking it and, in any case, fail to achieve it, having defined it in a way guaranteed to always place it just beyond our reach.

## THE POLITICS OF LIMITS— INTERESTS AND INTEREST GROUPS

Little I have said here is likely to commend itself to our present political way of life, one that looks to a constant improvement of health as a way to greater human fulfillment and the satisfying of many interests, social as well as economic. It is a way of life that joins together the language of progress, of freedom of choice, and of efficiency with a view of the body that only with the greatest reluctance concedes its limitations, its ultimate finitude. For politicians and legislators, this makes for a delicate, volatile combination. They must commend and work for progress and yet, at the same time, find ways to control the costs of medicine and its power to dominate other social needs. Public demand for better healthcare can be ferocious, and any proposals to cut back on or limit it can expect strong resistance, often stated in a way as to imply moral coldness and indifference to human suffering—or, even worse, as a form of involuntary euthanasia. That kind of pressure and intimidation should be resisted, and it can be expected that various interest groups will press vigorously for the claims of their constituents.

Many of the claims will be legitimate and understandable. That in itself will not necessarily show that they are affordable or, in light of other needs, of the highest priority. The principles developed in earlier chapters provide one set of criteria by which to measure such claims. Taken together they will, at the least, serve to dampen their insistence; and, taken individually, they may prove decisive in showing a claim to be poorly based.

In the face of demands for research to cure still more disease, or for money to extend the delivery of curative medicine, one can apply the principle of *sufficiency:* will it simply add to an already high level of general health, adding years to lives already long, or will it perhaps be of special value to achieve a greater *balance* for an age or economic group that falls below the common norm? Is it consistent with the principle of *symmetry*, that is, with the goal of developing only those forms of curative medicine that promise a good outcome, in both the short and the long run, and in particular does it avoid generating cures that simply leave chronic illness in their wake? If it is a matter of introducing a new technology, thus requiring assessment, what are the chances of it succeeding in doing what it's meant to do, and doing it well? And if it should succeed, is there a chance that it could be all too successful, significantly increasing the long-term cost of care and

introducing potentially harmful social and cultural consequences? If it is a form of curative medicine, will it have a societal
benefit? Or, if the benefit is mainly to individuals, can it be
shown that the public need for care and caring, or for public
health and preventive measures, has already sufficiently been
met to allow the use of resources for those individual interests?

These are the kinds of questions for legislators to press upon
interest groups—and the kinds of questions the public should
press upon legislators should they seem prone to support forms
of healthcare that respond to special interests before they take
steps to meet more general needs.[21] The most important question to be put to a legislator is: Will the proposed legislation be
a meaningful part of a coherent long-term strategy? If not, it
should be resisted. In particular, it will become especially important to resist incrementalist arguments. By that I mean that
common form of political argument which holds that it is better
to get at least part of what one wants than to stubbornly hold out
for a full program. This kind of compromise policy should now
be rejected. Its past fruits are now part of our present problems—
piecemeal programs and a chaotic system. Partial programs are
in fact likely, because of their added cost, to make it harder, not
easier, to add further more comprehensive programs later. The
1965 Medicare and Medicaid programs, thought to be a shrewd
step on the way to national health insurance, probably had just
the opposite effect, making it harder—because of the sharply
rising cost of the 1965 programs as the years went on—to make
a case for a full universal health insurance plan. The passage in
1988 of the catastrophic illness program as part of Medicare may
have made it all the less likely that a much more important
program, one providing for good long-term care, will be able to
get through Congress in the near future. Mandated insurance
coverage, popular with state legislatures, is another similarly
poor approach. It requires coverage for specific treatments or
conditions in response to interest-group pressure, reflects no
systematic overall healthcare strategy, and creates burdens for
business and insurance companies that are often unfair and
insupportable.

# EVALUATING UNIVERSAL HEALTH INSURANCE PROPOSALS

The most appropriate and coherent way to deal with the problem of interest groups and piecemeal reform efforts would be some form of universal, national health insurance, a point now widely accepted (if not by politicians, at least by much of the healthcare community). It is the only way likely to be able to deal, at one and the same time, with the joint problems of inefficiency and inequity. How should we judge such proposals? By what criteria might they best be evaluated? Their potential to cope with inefficiency and inequity is one obvious test, and the proposals so far advanced primarily address themselves to those demands.

Yet there should also be a more severe demand, of great importance for the long run. How well do the various proposals address the basic and structural forces that have driven up the costs of and demand for healthcare? How well, that is, can they cope with the long-term health-demand pressures? If they fail to have some strategy for doing that, then any enacted plan will contain the seeds of its own destruction. If we are poised as a society to introduce some form of universal health insurance, a historically important step, then that should be done with an eye to the future, not just to immediate problems. It must, in that respect, have a way of coping with our deepest values and way of life, for it is those values which have created many of our present problems and will continue to wreak havoc in the future unless soon changed in important respects.

I will briefly review some of the leading proposals for universal coverage.[22] Uwe Reinhardt has proposed what he calls a "fail-safe health-insurance system." Its principal feature would be a federal program that would automatically cover any person without adequate private coverage, and which would be paid for by excise taxes and by a general income tax surcharge. It would require that those covered by the program receive their (nonemergency) care through an HMO or some other managed-care system. Those systems would competitively bid for the right to serve the federally insured patients. Reinhardt has estimated that the additional cost of such a program would be between $10 billion and $15 billion a year. Alain Enthoven and Richard Kronick have proposed a system that would also rely upon managed-care plans, with those plans competing with each other for contracts with employers or state-level "public sponsors." It would be paid for by a combination of employer-mandated coverage and increased income tax. They estimate that it would require an additional $12.8 billion of federal expenditures (and $12.4 billion in additional taxes), and would increase total healthcare expenditures by $15 billion—a one-time increase, they say, thereafter stabilized by restraint in the growth of healthcare costs.

In a bill first introduced by Senators Edward Kennedy and Lowell Weicker in 1987, the proposal is to require that all employers provide a basic minimum package of health insurance for their full-time workers. It would stimulate the creation of regional insurers who would competitively bid to provide low-cost insurance to small businesses, those which would be most burdened by an employer-based plan. Its overall costs have not been well calculated, but the Congressional Budget Office estimated that it would result initially in an addition of $300 million to the annual overall federal deficit. Still another strategy has been pursued by some states, that of creating health insurance pools, and the state of Massachusetts has initiated a plan that will place a heavy burden on employers, with some general tax assistance, to provide care. A proposal advanced by the National Leadership Commission on Health Care would use a combination of incentives to encourage stronger employer coverage and various individual and employer fees to provide coverage for the indigent. I would mention, finally, a proposal, the "National Health Program," by a group of physicians. It is the one proposal that would eventually turn the entire health insurance problem over to the federal government, aiming to cover every person in the country under a single, comprehensive national health insurance program. Its authors believe that, with the savings it would make possible, it would not significantly add to present healthcare costs.

What should we look for as proposals of this kind are debated in the years ahead? Those plans that would place a greater burden upon employers, and build upon competition for healthcare contracts, probably have more political feasibility than those which would create a single federal system of insurance, though the latter would probably more effectively control costs. I want to focus, however, on a different consideration. Each of the plans assumes that greater efficiency can solve our problem of healthcare—that we can dampen supply by forcing those who provide care to do so as efficiently as possible in order to be competitive, and that we can dampen demand by requiring consumers to be more cost conscious. They do not address the problem of the structural dynamic underlying the pressure for healthcare and the increase in costs—that of an aging society, commitment to medical progress, and public demand. Only public demand is given any attention, but even then not in its inherent features but only in the formal language of using market forces to restrict demand. The Enthoven-Kronich plan, for example, ultimately rests on the belief "that competition to serve cost-conscious purchasers [through managed-care plans] could motivate cost-reducing innovations and slow the growth of healthcare spending."[23] They rely for their economic efficacy on "requiring consumers to be conscious of costs in choosing among healthcare organizations."[24] For its part, the physicians' proposal believes that its savings will come from reduced bureaucracy, improved planning, and the ability to establish overall spending limits.[25]

If proposals of this kind are to have a long-term value, then they must find a way to expand their scope and encompass the deeper questions of entitlements and our way of life. Why is this necessary? Because all solutions that look to efficiency evade the central problem: How are we to set limits on our aspirations, restrict the frontiers of progress, and find a sensible place for health among our other societal needs? What are managed-care systems to do about new, expensive, but clearly effective technologies? What will they do about AIDS? What are they to do about the costs of long-term care, which will grow as the number and proportion of elderly grow?[26] The proposal of a financing mechanism, without parallel proposals about ways to change our fundamental values in some important respects, only meets part of the problem. To assume that we can simply solve our problems by forcing people to make "cost-conscious" choices, or to live with federal limits, is a thin and fragile solution at best unless accompanied by a fresh understanding of the place of health in our lives, and of the meaning and place of medical advancement. How are we supposed to think through the making of such choices, and to come to some satisfying and viable understanding of the content of those decisions? Without that understanding, we will—if externally imposed pressure itself is supposed to do the job—become enraged, or simply keep increasing the overall outlay on healthcare to stay one jump ahead of angry rebellion. The very success of these plans, or any like them, requires that we change the very context and content of the public discussion. Otherwise, even if we get them, they will probably disintegrate after a few years. We will be back where we started, only more cynical and angry.

The issue is not simply to get people to be more conscious of the costs of their choices, or to be prepared to make some difficult choices. That they can be forced to do. The underlying issue is also to know what would count as wise and good choices, and to know just what choices it is best to have in the first place. Those questions cannot be well answered in social isolation by individuals, or well posed by the society that lays them upon individuals, without some common and sustained grappling with the way, in the context of constraints, we should come to understand our human condition in the face of illness and death. To give people a "choice" about such matters of ultimate importance is wonderful; they should have it. But to give them a choice without an accompanying profound societal effort to think together about the meaning and value of health, about the desire to cure illness and hold off death, about what they genuinely need for their real well-being, about the obligations that should bind people together—to give them a choice, that is, in a cultural vacuum (or, just as bad, in a cultural context that continues to cherish the values of choice, progress, and the denial of limits)—would be to create a new system still infected with the virus that brought down the old one.

We desperately need a universal health insurance plan, one that makes a decent level of healthcare available to all. We no less desperately need a new set of values to accompany it. The one without the other will be useless, badly missing the point of our present crisis, which is moral and not just economic.

# CHAPTER 8

# TO KILL AND TO RATION: PRESERVING THE DIFFERENCE

One of the great and perennial problems of medicine is knowing how best to respond to the ragged edge of progress, that historically ever-changing, ever-evolving point where sickness and health, life and death, come roughly and irregularly together. The conventional response has been to ignore its permanent reality, working ceaselessly to overcome one ragged edge and then move to the next, and then the next, and then the next again. That is a hopeless venture, at least in the pursuit of individual cure. We cannot ultimately overcome the ragged edge, and no degree of efficiency will make it economically rational to remain on our present course of relentless and uncritical medical progress. The more successful that progress, the more of it we want, and the more of it we want, the more economically insupportable it becomes.

Yet what if we could agree on the credibility of that contention? What if we could then come to curtail our long-standing efforts to overcome the ragged edge, to accept more illness and death than we are now inclined to do? What would we, should we, come to think about, and do about, those people—real, identifiable, needy, and desperate—who are on the present ragged edge, suffering from a not-yet-curable cancer, or liver failure, or heart disease, or genetic defect? That thought is, and should be, painful. For we know full well that edge might be moved forward, probably could be, if we just carried out more research, or invested more in better technology or facilities, or worked harder to improve our early-warning diagnostic techniques. Our imagination of the people on that edge, who may be our parents or spouses or children or dear friends or of course ourselves, makes us reluctant to simply tolerate, to passively accept—however great our caring—the ragged edge and not to do anything about it.

Yet we are reaching the point where we will have to do just that. Could we learn to live with that imagination, ever tugging at our compassion for others, ever pulling for that matter at our own fear of mortality? We might well concede as a general and abstract proposition that we cannot afford limitless progress, even concede its ultimate folly, but that is not the same as accepting with moral equanimity the consequences of such a disavowal, which are suffering and death. Can we find a way of accommodating those consequences with honor and integrity?[1]

I want to get at that problem by examining the movement to legalize active euthanasia and assisted suicide. It poses issues that transcend the immediate euthanasia debate and touch upon matters of direct concern to our understanding of health and its place in our lives. The primary argument for active euthanasia and assisted suicide has always been a relatively simple one. A dying person, or one whose life has become intolerably burdensome, has the right to request to have his or her life directly ended by another if that is necessary to avoid suffering or a hopelessly compromised existence.[2] Alternatively, we should, with the help of others, be enabled to kill ourselves to achieve the same end. The popular phrase "mercy killing" refers to the killing of one person by another as an act of kindness, not as an act of malice or self-interest on the part of the one who does the killing (or assists in a suicide). It is often said that we have a right to this kind of mercy. On what grounds? The moral foundation of this claimed right is that our body is our own, and that our life should be subject to our self-determination. We have, it is said, a right to end our own life. If we cannot accomplish this on our own, another person may, with our permission, end it for us as an act of compassion. The law, it is argued, should recognize and sanction this possibility, with suitable procedures and safeguards to ensure a serious reason for doing so and to validate the voluntary nature of the decision.

The proposed legalization of active euthanasia and assisted suicide is important to the allocation issue for a number of reasons. It offers for many an alternative approach to the problem of scarcity and the prospect of rationing. If we would simply allow people to be able to end their lives when they voluntarily chose to do so, it is said, we could simultaneously enhance self-determination and the conservation of resources. The well-known fact that a small minority of patients, particularly those at the end of life, consume a disproportionately large share of resources is, it has also been urged, a powerful reason to move in that direction. It is a solution that would nicely combine autonomy and efficiency, the two deepest values behind the belief in medical progress. Others resist any move in that direction. There is a deep concern among some that the drive for efficiency and cost containment will become (if it has not already become) a cloak behind which to rid ourselves of the costly and burdensome, especially those who are the most vulnerable and powerless, the least useful and "productive."[3] How are we morally to distinguish between the allocation of scarce resources and involuntary euthanasia, both of which have a similar outcome, a loss of life?

There is still another reason for considering allocation and euthanasia together in the context of this book. The moral logic of active euthanasia and assisted suicide rests on much the same premise as that of the entire enterprise of high-technology curative medicine: the desire, the demand, the claimed right of human beings to fight against, to master and to control, illness and death. The struggle I have sketched between a priority of cure and a priority of care brings us squarely back to that issue, at the center of the most important choice that the need to better manage our healthcare system ultimately presents. How hard and in what ways should we struggle against our mortality, and what should we do when we lose that struggle? The question of active euthanasia and assisted suicide, then, provides a window through which to look at a basic issue raised by efforts to think about the place of health and illness in our lives and to devise a good system of healthcare.

## EXPANDING CHOICE AND SAVING MONEY: THE EUTHANASIA DEBATE

Why does the interest in active euthanasia and assisted suicide seem to have taken on a renewed vitality of late? It is hardly a new topic, going back to Greek and Roman classical culture. More recently, it has had some zealous supporters in Great Britain, since the mid- to late-nineteenth century, and in this country since early in the twentieth. As far back as the 1930s it was debated in a few state legislatures, and bills were introduced to legalize it, always unsuccessfully. But until the past few years it was never a powerful or widespread movement. It is quite possible, indeed, that it is still not as potent as it may seem on the surface, as suggested by the defeat of a well-publicized 1988 California referendum initiative.[4] Still, there does seem evidence of new stirrings in this country, and the situation in Holland—where it is legally tolerated and openly practiced—represents a prominent and visible case of change in a country with values much like ours.[5] What is going on?

The most plausible answer is that the interest in euthanasia represents the confluence of two powerful forces, one medical and one cultural. There is the power of medicine to extend life under poor circumstances, now widely and increasingly feared. That power invokes the dread of a death tortuously and aggressively extended by tubes and machines, or drawn out for months or years in a nursing home in a haze of debilitation and dementia. While this feared picture is in some respects a caricature, it is not without foundation. Since the 1960s, death has been an institutional event, with over 80 percent of deaths occurring in hospitals. Even those dying in nursing homes are likely, in an acute crisis, to be taken to a hospital. Hospitals themselves have become different institutions, more than ever oriented to intensive care. When a patient dies in a hospital it is increasingly the result of some conscious decision to stop aggressive life-saving efforts, vivid evidence of a medical power able to give almost every patient at least a few more hours or days. Patients are as a rule put on respirators more quickly than was the case twenty years ago, and they are much more likely to be fed artificially should their frailty or dementia render them incapable or uninterested in eating (and new methods of artificial nutrition and hydration have made it easier to do so).

Along with these technological and institutional changes has been the powerful individualism of our society, which asserts our right to autonomy, to be the master of our own fate, to be in control of our bodies. While always part of the American tradition (as noted long ago by de Tocqueville), the 1960s and 1970s saw that individualism vigorously extended into the medical system. The patient's rights movement, the centrality given autonomy in recent medical ethics, and court decisions upholding patient self-determination reflect that development. The combined power, moreover, of a deeply philosophical and religious tradition of respect for individual life and a medical tradition powerfully oriented to treatment and the preservation of life creates what too often seems an uncontrollable momentum toward relentless, aggressive, unthinking treatment, usually for the best of motives. How is control to be regained in the face of this confluence of forces? For many the answer seems obvious and unavoidable, that of active euthanasia and assisted suicide.

Public-opinion surveys surely register a sharp shift in that direction. Comparative Louis Harris surveys show that 53 percent of respondents in 1973 opposed active euthanasia (with 37 percent favorable), while by 1985 61 percent were favorable, with only 36 percent opposed.[6] These changes in public opinion, it should be noted, closely parallel recent changes in medical practice and patterns of medical care. The proliferation of more sophisticated high-technology care and a rising worry about malpractice suits and criminal indictments among physicians and hospital administrators were all taking place during this same period. Almost everyone could, by the end of the 1970s, think of someone close to them personally whose life had seemed to be drawn out past any point of benefit or common sense. Another development was coming to be noticed as well. By the early 1980s some 30 to 35 percent of Medicare expenditures were devoted to that 5 percent of the total number of recipients who were in their last year of life, and similarly provocative figures were emerging about the cost of care for the dying and critically ill in all age groups.[7] Since many of those people did not, presumably, want all the life-extending treatment they received, it has been contended that to give them a greater choice, the right to say no, would save considerable money.

## EUTHANASIA: ECONOMICS AND SELF-DETERMINATION

I turn first to the belief that active euthanasia would save money. Of course since it has not been legal, we have no historical basis to make valid cost projections. We can only make some guesses, working with the evidence we now have about efforts to increase the right of patients to ask for a termination of their treatment, to be allowed to die. Based on that evidence, however, there are no solid grounds to believe that moving one step further, to active euthanasia, would make any decisive economic difference. Some thirty-eight states have in recent years enacted "living will" or "natural death" acts to make possible advanced directives, that is, the empowering of people to specify the conditions under which they would have life-extending treatment stopped. There is no evidence from any of those states that such legislation has reduced costs. Nor is there any evidence either, on closer inspection, that the money spent on the elderly in the last year of their life is demonstrably wasteful. The most elderly and debilitated patients, it turns out, do not receive the most expensive high-technology care in any case (though there is a strong trend of the extension of advanced technological medicine from younger to older patients).[8] As for the other dying elderly it was not necessarily known in advance that they were actually dying. The art of medical prognostication is still poorly developed (and the most expensive patients turn out to be those expected to die but who in fact survived).[9]

I am not claiming here that giving people more choice about the manner of their dying could not and will not save money. I am only claiming that there is as yet no *good evidence* that it will, or that it could happen to the extent necessary to make a *decisive* economic difference for the healthcare system as a whole. That would require savings of tens of billions of dollars. No doubt the addition of active euthanasia as an option would make some additional difference. Yet to envision savings of a significant kind must remain a great act of faith, much too great to be seen as a solution to the problem of costly life-saving medical treatment. At best, predictions in this direction should be restrained. Some savings, yes; great savings, no.

A few simple observations should tell us why restraint of expectations in that direction is in order. As fast as we find a way to save money in one direction, we typically add new technological innovations in another, or (as in the case of the elderly) find a new population on whom to deploy existing technologies. While most people, moreover, seem to agree with the principle that treatment should be stopped when it does no more good (a notion hard to oppose), almost everyone might choose more treatment if there was some promise of some success. But that is just what medical progress always seems to offer, some promise of some success; and that is why, when there is doubt (as there almost always can be), treatment continues. As Jessica Muller and Barbara Koenig have noted in an unusually perceptive study of physician practices in the care of the dying: "The patient is not even defined as dying until the clinicians determine that there are no further interventions they can make that will improve the patient's condition . . . acknowledgement of a patient's dying status may not be made until death is imminent or, in some cases, has already occurred."[10]

The problem, I have come to think, is not the last illness, about which we can usually find agreement. The real problem is that of the penultimate illness, the one that—our doctors and families and our own will to live assure us—is not actually our last illness, however much it may look like it. If we will only keep trying, one more time . . . just one. In each patient the story of medical progress can be acted out once again, and as we know it is the nature of that story to want almost always to have another chapter.

If the likely savings from greater self-determination to the point of euthanasia in one's dying or incurable illness are at best uncertain, the moral question of that self-determination raises still more complex problems and of a different order. Two contentions in particular have gained ground in recent years, and they have lent an air of reasonableness to the drive for active euthanasia that has cracked what had otherwise for some years been a stale, and more or less stalemated, intellectual debate. One of them is a revitalized argument for autonomy, pushing the idea of a right to self-determination as far as it can go, to the right to be killed on request. The other is the claim that the traditional distinction between killing and allowing to die, commission and omission, is simply wrong.

What is the status of the self-determination argument? That question is best answered by looking briefly at the main traditions that have opposed euthanasia. One of them is clearly religious. Its foundation is the belief that God alone is the author of our life and that, whatever other rights we may have, the right to take or destroy our own life is not among them. This general conviction remains strong in many religious groups, and explains the profound reluctance of many to terminate treatment. This conviction has not manifested an indifference to human pain and suffering; indeed, religious groups have been historically among those most concerned to provide healthcare and to relieve suffering. It has expressed, instead, a belief that our life is simply not our own, but God's.[11] The other dominant tradition has focused on the potentially harmful consequences of legalizing euthanasia.[12] This tradition, more secular in its origins, has been willing in the hands of some of its proponents to grant that, strictly taken, we may indeed have a right to have our life ended to relieve our pain. Yet while there can thus be some morally acceptable reasons in some cases for euthanasia, it would be a great mistake to legalize it as a practice. That would invite, indeed court, misuse.

This secular tradition has heavily depended upon speculations about the consequences of making euthanasia legal, that it could quickly get out of hand and lead to deadly abuse. But that argument is necessarily problematic, mainly because the speculation, even if intuitively reasonable, rests on no clear historical evidence that abuse must always and necessarily follow legalization; there are no modern historical precedents to observe. The Nazi experience is only partially relevant. There was, to be sure, a strong movement in the years prior to the Nazi regime to hold that some lives are "not worth living," and should not be sustained, and that may well have contributed a poisonous background condition that made the Nazi atrocities more likely.[13] But, strictly speaking, the Nazis did not move from legal voluntary euthanasia to involuntary killing. They never had the first phase at all—theirs was hardly a regime strong on self-determination and the right to control one's body—but went straight to the killing. With the danger of involuntary euthanasia in mind, however, it has been contended that carefully drawn laws could make abuse difficult and hazardous, punishable by heavy penalties.

We do not, in any case, know exactly what the hazards of a legalization of euthanasia would mean (though I am among those who would fear the worst). But one can much more confidently predict that the greater the fear of medicine in our dying, the greater the willingness there will be to venture those hazards. They may well seem the lesser evils. For just that reason, a more potent argument against euthanasia is needed, one that is not exclusively dependent upon uncertain legal and social consequences but can show the intrinsic wrongfulness of euthanasia.

I will sketch, but not fully detail, such an argument.[14] It is, first, a mistake to classify active euthanasia and assisted suicide as acts solely expressive of individual autonomy, as is now common. On the contrary, because they entail the assistance of another (someone who will kill us in the case of active euthanasia, or help us kill ourselves in the case of assisted suicide), they are essentially a form of concerted communal action, even though the community in question may only be two people. That ceases to make them individual acts; they become a form of social action. Second, we have never allowed killing as a form of a contractual relationship between two consenting adults. The killing of another is now justified only in cases of self-defense, capital punishment, and just war. In none of those cases is the killing for the benefit of the person killed, but allowed only to protect the lives or welfare of others, even if that life is our own (as in self-defense). There must, in short, be a public interest at stake in the taking of life. We have otherwise considered it too great a power to be given to individuals to serve their private ends, even if they be good ends. Third, even if I could make a case that I have a right to self-determination even unto death, it does not follow that my right to kill myself can be transformed into the right of someone else to kill me. What is the basis of his right to do so? My authorization? But what right have I to authorize another to kill?

An analogy suggests itself. Why has the central liberal tradition of self-determination consistently excluded the right to voluntarily become the slave of another? John Stuart Mill, in his classic work "On Liberty," provided a compelling reason. "By selling himself for a slave," he wrote," [a person] abdicates his liberty; he forgoes any future use of it beyond that single act. . . . The principle of freedom cannot require that he should be free not to be free. It is not freedom to be allowed to alienate his freedom."[15] The same reasoning can extend to that alienation both of freedom and of life represented by euthanasia; it is a double alienation. I would add to that another reason. Just as there should be a limit on our power to alienate our life and freedom because of what it forces us to cede to another, it cannot be a good for those given the power to enslave or kill us. No human being, whatever the motives, should have that kind of ultimate power over the fate of another. It is to give away precisely that which makes us human, our freedom and life, and to give to another that which they should not have, power over the freedom and life of another. It takes too much from ourselves and gives too much to another. It is also to create the wrong kind of relationship between people, the creation of a community that sanctions private killings between its members. Even if we fully grant the argument that acts of euthanasia stemming from compassion and mercy can embody some commendable aspects, they are not sufficient to justify so momentous a social change, one that would be fundamental and far-reaching in its implications for human relationships. It would be to make the killing of another a matter of individual choice and personal contract rather than societal judgment and (rarely invoked) social necessity.

## KILLING AND ALLOWING TO DIE

If a lessened worry about the consequences of legal euthanasia has been gaining ground, there has been an even more powerful challenge to the traditional prohibition. No distinction, many now argue, can be made between killing and allowing to die, or between an act of commission and one of omission.[16] The traditional distinction between them rests on the commonplace observation that lives can come to an end as the result of (a) the direct action of another who becomes the cause of death (as in shooting a person) and (b) the result of impersonal forces where no human agent has acted (death by lightning, or by disease). The purpose of the distinction has been to separate those deaths caused by human action and those caused by nonhuman events. It is, as a distinction, meant to say something about human beings and their relationship to the world. It is a way of articulating the difference between those actions for which human beings can be held rightly responsible, or blamed, and those of which they are innocent. At issue is the difference between physical causality, the realm of impersonal events, and moral culpability, the realm of human responsibility.

Little imagination is required to see how the distinction between killing and allowing to die can be challenged. The standard objection encompasses two points. The first is that people can become equally dead by our omissions as well as our commissions. We can refrain from saving them when it is possible to do so, and they will be just as dead as if we had shot them. It is our decision itself that is the reason for their death, not necessarily how we effectuate that decision. That contention establishes the basis of the second point. If we *intend* their death, it can be brought about as well by omitted acts as by those we commit. The crucial moral point is not how they die, but our intention about their death. We can, then, be responsible for the death of another by intending that they die and accomplishing that end by standing aside and allowing them to die.

Despite these criticisms—resting upon ambiguities that can readily be acknowledged—the distinction between killing and allowing to die remains valid. It has not only a logical validity but, no less importantly, a social validity whose place must be as central in moral judgments about allocation as in individual patient decisions. As a way of putting the distinction into perspective, I want to propose that it is best understood as expressing three different, though overlapping, perspectives on nature and human action. I will call them the metaphysical, the moral, and the medical perspectives.

## Metaphysical

The first and most fundamental premise of the distinction between killing and allowing to die is that there is a sharp difference between the self and the external world. Unlike the childish fantasy that the world is nothing more than a projection of the self, or the neurotic person's fear that he or she is responsible for everything that goes wrong, the distinction is meant to uphold a simple notion: There is a world external to the self that has its own, and independent, causal dynamism. The mistake behind a conflation of killing and allowing to die is to assume that the self has become master of everything within and outside of the self. It is as if the conceit that modern man might ultimately control nature has been internalized—that if the self might be able to influence nature by its actions, then the self and nature must be one.

That is a fantasy. The fact that we can intervene in nature, and cure or control many diseases, does not erase the difference between the self and the external world. It is as "out there" as ever, even if more under our sway. That sway, however great, is always limited. We can cure disease, but not always the chronic illness that comes with the cure. We can forestall death with modern medicine, but death always wins in the long run because of the limitations of the body, inherently and stubbornly beyond final human control. We can distinguish between a diseased body and an aging body, but in the end they always become one and the same body. To attempt to deny the distinction between killing and allowing to die is, then, to mistakenly impute more power to human action than it actually has and to accept the conceit that nature has now fallen wholly within the realm of human control. Nothing could be further from the truth.

## Moral

At the center of the distinction between killing and allowing to die is the difference between physical causality and moral culpability. To bring the life of another to an end by an injection is to directly kill the other. Our action is the physical cause of the death. To allow someone to die from a disease we cannot cure (and that we did not cause) is to permit the disease to act as the cause of death. The notion of physical causality in both cases rests on the distinction between human agency and the action of external nature. The ambiguity arises precisely because we can be morally culpable for killing someone (if we have no moral right to do so, as we would in self-defense) and no less culpable for allowing someone to die (if we have both the possibility and the obligation of keeping that person alive). Thus there are cases where, morally speaking, it makes no difference whether we killed or allowed to die. We are equally responsible morally. In those cases, the lines of physical causality and moral culpability happen to cross. Yet the fact that they can cross in some cases in no way shows that they are always, or even usually, one and the same. We can ordinarily find the difference in all but the most obscure cases. We should not, then, use the ambiguity of such cases to do away altogether with the distinction between killing and allowing to die. The ambiguity may obscure, but does not erase, the line between the two.

There is one group of cases that is especially troublesome. Even if we grant the ordinary validity between killing and allowing to die, what about those cases that combine (a) an illness that renders a patient unable to carry out an ordinary biological function (to eat or breathe on his own, for example) and (b) we then turn off a respirator or remove an artificial feeding tube? On the level of physical causality, have we killed the patient or allowed him to die? In one sense, it is our action that shortens his life, and yet in another sense it is his underlying disease that brings his life to an end. I believe it reasonable to say that, since his life was being sustained by artificial means (respirator or tube), and that was necessary because of the fact that he had an incapacitating disease, his disease is the ultimate reality behind his death. But for that reality, there would be no need for artificial sustenance in the first place and no moral issue at all. To lose sight of the paramount reality of the disease is to lose sight of the difference between our selves and the outer world. It is surely true, as Dan Brock has put it, that "but for" our action in removing a feeding tube, the patient would not have died when he did. Yet I think it even more importantly true that he would not have been at risk of death at all "but for" his disease. It is the ultimately decisive reality, the one that sets into motion whatever follows.[17]

I quickly add, and underscore, a moral point. The person who turns off a respirator or pulls a feeding tube will be morally culpable if there is not a good reason to do so. That the patient has been allowed to die of his underlying condition does not morally excuse the one who omitted those actions. The moral question is whether we are obliged to continue treating a life that is being artificially sustained, and that will depend on the circumstances of that life. To cease treatment may or may not be morally acceptable—but it should be understood, in either case, that the ultimate occasion of death was the underlying disease, now no longer resisted.

There is an analogous issue of importance. Physicians frequently feel far more responsible morally for stopping the use of a life-saving device than for not using it in the first place. While the psychology behind that feeling may be understandable, it is now almost universally denied that there is any moral difference of significance, as such, between withholding treatment and withdrawing treatment.[18] The point of the denial is precisely that an intervention into a disease process does not erase the underlying disease. To accept the fact that a disease cannot be controlled after an effort has been made to do so, and treatment is then stopped, is as morally acceptable as deciding in advance that it cannot successfully be controlled. The distinction between withholding and withdrawing should be rejected for the same reason that the distinction between killing and allowing to die should be maintained, to keep clearly before us the external reality and independent causality of disease.

## Medical

A major social purpose of the distinction between killing and allowing to die has been that of protecting the historical role of the physician as one who tries to cure or comfort patients rather than to kill them. It is to help keep clear the difference between what disease does (kill) and what physicians try to do (cure and heal). Physicians have been given special knowledge about the body, and knowledge that can be used to kill or to cure.

Physicians are also given great privileges in making use of that knowledge, ordinarily free of day-to-day oversight. It is thus all the more important that their social role and power be, and be seen to be, a limited power. It may be used only to cure or comfort, never to kill. They have not been given, nor should they be given, the power to use their knowledge and skills to bring life to an end. That kind of power would introduce a fundamental ambiguity in their role. It would open the way for powerful misuse and, no less importantly, represent an intrinsic violation of what it has historically meant to be a physician.[19]

Yet if it is possible for physicians to misuse their knowledge and power in order to directly kill people, are they thereby required to use that same knowledge always to keep people alive, always to resist a disease that can itself kill the patient? The traditional answer has been, not necessarily. For the physician's ultimate obligation is to the welfare of the patient, and excessive treatment can be as detrimental to that welfare as inadequate treatment. Put another way, the obligation to resist the lethal power of disease is limited. It ceases when the patient is unwilling to have the disease resisted, or when the resistance no longer serves the patient's welfare. Behind this moral premise is the recognition that disease (of some kind) ultimately triumphs and that death is inevitable sooner or later; death is not, in any case, always the greatest human evil. In practice, however, this insight is often ignored.

I suggested earlier that the most potent motive at present for active euthanasia and assisted suicide is that of a dread of the power of medicine. That power seems to take on a drive of its own regardless of the welfare or wishes of patients. No one can easily say no—not physicians, not patients, not families. That happens because too many physicians, ironically, have already come to believe that it is their choice, and their choice alone, which brings about death. They do not want to exercise that kind of authority and thus they continue to treat, feeling that if they do not do so they will be causally and morally responsible for the death. They have been put in what seems to them an impossible situation. The solution to their problem is to underscore the validity and importance of the distinction between killing and allowing to die; and the latter is not the former. They cannot be made ultimately responsible for what disease and mortality do to people.

## RATIONING AND INVOLUNTARY EUTHANASIA

The euthanasia and rationing debates are easily likely to mutually confuse, even pollute, each other. To avoid that, it is necessary to be clear about the difference between directly killing a known patient and making an allocation decision whose effect will be to allow someone to die who might otherwise be saved. How can it be morally plausible to condemn the one but allow the other? The answer depends upon understanding that, in the face of scarcity and to advance other societal goods, no society is required to devote an unreasonable or harmful share of its resources to the struggle against illness and disease. Disease is part of the reality of human nature and biology and should be struggled against in prudent ways only. To allow disease finally to triumph is not a wrongful act if that comes at the end of reasonable efforts to resist it; and an unlimited effort can be unreasonable. But let me look more carefully at the relationship between the euthanasia and allocation debates.

I have tried to argue why the traditional prohibition of direct killing has been correct: active euthanasia runs the risk of corruption and wrongly extends to another the right to control our bodies. But the strongest challenge to the tradition of late has been a denial that there is a meaningful distinction to be made between killing and allowing to die, or between an act of commission and one of omission. While this challenge has come most strongly from those favoring the legalization of active euthanasia, it has seemed to draw at least implicit support from some pro-life groups as well, opposed to euthanasia. For the former, their argument is that if there is no serious distinction to be drawn between killing and allowing to die, then our present acceptance of allowing to die ought to be extended to active killing when death is morally justifiable and desirable. This is especially defensible when such killing would actually be more merciful and simultaneously make a helpful financial contribution as well. For the latter, while there may be a strictly logical distinction between the two, "allowing to die" is a slogan that has come to be used as a legitimizing rationale to end the life of those who are burdensome or judged to have lives not worth living.[20] Since active killing is to be rejected, we should also be highly suspicious of the concept of allowing to die, and no less suspicious of contentions that a shortage of resources requires that some people be allowed to die in the name of economic savings.

This challenge, from the liberal and the conservative sides simultaneously, promises maximum confusion. It will make it that much harder to have careful discussions of the euthanasia issue and all but impossible to have a coherent consideration of the allocation problem. If the implications of doing away with the distinction between killing and allowing to die are momentous for the euthanasia debate, and the treatment of individual patients, they are equally grave for the allocation debate. It is hard, in fact, to see how we can have a sensible allocation debate without upholding the validity of the distinction. Without it, we face a number of stark alternatives. If we cannot morally distinguish between killing and allowing to die, then every allocation decision can be construed as a decision to allow some people to die and thus would be the same as directly killing those people. A refusal to provide life-saving coverage under an entitlement program will be seen as not simply active euthanasia, but active *involuntary* euthanasia, a direct killing of people without their consent.[21] A decision to allocate money, say, to education rather than to healthcare will be seen as a decision to kill people for the sake of education (more specifically, to kill the sick to help children).

Given that understanding, health needs would ordinarily trump all other social claims. Any other choice would be seen as cruel. I do not invoke here a hypothetical worry. Even now, those who have tried to limit health allocations have been accused by some of using financial arguments as a covert way of ridding society of people unwanted on other grounds, or simply thought too burdensomely expensive to be worth support.[22] Others have been no less quick to complain that for a society to deny health resources to the needy, or to want to limit an entitlement program, is a selfish way to keep for itself resources that would save human lives, a murderous course.

I believe that way of thinking, whether from right or left, is misleading and harmful. To first deny the distinction between killing and allowing to die, and then to use that denial as a way of circumventing a necessary allocation debate or decision, adds a social error to a metaphysical one. But to say this is not to deny that allocation decisions have important life and death implications, or that some allocation decisions can be used to mask abominable moral attitudes or practices, or that some allocation decisions can be wrong and unfair. I am only trying, at this point, to say that issues of that kind must be decided on their own merits, and not dealt with by being confused with, or ignoring, the distinction between killing and allowing to die. That helps nothing.

But how, then, can we make difficult allocation decisions in ways that avoid any taint of using them as a way of wrongly killing people? I want to try to answer this question at two levels, first that of politics and procedure, and then by considering the more profound issue lying beneath it, that of the extent to which we should, as a society, struggle against our mortality and elevate control over illness and death to a position of supreme importance.

If we believe that it is the obligation of the healthcare system as a whole to meet each and every individual curative need, allowing desire and demand and research and scientific possibility to determine what counts as need, then this will be a hopeless and fruitless task. If we, moreover, believe that the demand of justice is that each and every individual have an equal opportunity to take advantage of what will meet his or her curative need, then it will not be possible to meet that demand. No government can any longer do that, especially in the face of constantly expanding technological possibilities. It will, in fact, be hazardous to many other important societal needs to even make the attempt. A more reasonable, and feasible, alternative is that of meeting the individual need for care and caring (guaranteed to all by government), then through other government or private programs of insurance going a reasonable but limited distance toward meeting curative needs, and finally leaving to the market the meeting of those claimed needs beyond the capacity of institutional and entitlement mechanisms.

With this model of a healthcare system in mind, fairness and equity can be defined as follows. First, the ultimate test of a healthcare system cannot be whether each and every person has an equal opportunity to live an equally long life in equally good health; that is an impossible goal. It is, instead, whether some reasonable minimal level of individual need has been met, not the guaranteed opportunity for some maximal level. Giving a priority to caring, and to vigorous public health and health-promotion programs, could achieve that level. Second, in going beyond that minimal level, the provision by government (and related social mechanisms) of some further level of individuated curative medicine should rest on principles and procedures of a kind designed to balance the entire range of societal needs, not simply health alone. The principles of *sufficiency* (adequate societal health in general) and *symmetry* (coherence between length of life and quality of life) are means toward that end. Third, there should be a constant effort to see to it that no significant social group—particularly age and socioeconomic groups—falls significantly short of its share relative to other groups.

If those three conditions were met, there would be no grounds for a charge that the healthcare system was one engaged in tacit involuntary euthanasia, or that it was singling out the weak, the powerless, or the unproductive for special, murderous discrimination. It is not necessary for the system to cure the illness or save the life of every individual to avoid the charge of involuntary euthanasia or unjust allocation. That charge would be justified only if the system failed in an ongoing and patterned way to take account of the needs of particular groups,

leaving them outside of the system or leaving them disproportionately short of that to which most others have access.

## CONTROL, EUTHANASIA, AND ALLOCATION

Yet there remains an abiding dilemma inherent in developing a
healthcare system in the company of an aging society, technological progress, and expansive public demand. If we believe it a
basic human right to seek without limit or restraint to overcome
illness and death—to decisively control our bodily fate—and to
make use of scientific knowledge and technological prowess
to do so, then we will *inevitably* move in a direction certain to
outstrip our resources and distort our overall social priorities.
That much our present course is revealing to us (despite persistent efforts to convince ourselves that greater efficiency would
make it possible). If, by contrast, we believe that it is fitting in the
name of other societal goods to limit our drive and our aspirations for improved health, and thus also our healthcare resources, we seem to be resigning ourselves to a course close to an
old-fashioned fatalism. That course means, it would seem, an
acceptance of avoidable suffering and death, dooming those on
the present ragged edge, on the frontier of individual need, to a
death that need not be theirs.

It is this latter course we must risk. We cannot avoid it. We
should not be intimidated by charges that to rein in the pursuit
of health progress will mean, to use the favorite cliché, "turning
back the clock," and be unfair or cruel to those who will become
ill and die as a result of our omissions. The charge of fatalism can
be rejected out of hand. We have already achieved enormous
progress, and already live, and will continue to live, extraordinarily healthy lives by any historical standard. We are not necessarily likely to make ourselves notably happier or more
satisfied with life by adding indefinitely more health to it. We are
more likely only to increase the level of our dissatisfaction, and
we will certainly increase our financial strain. We have already
reached a point of diminishing returns on the satisfaction that

improved general health can bring. We need a healthcare system that can learn better how to meet the abiding human need for care, develop moderate and feasible aspirations for cure, and come to see the value of living within restricted frontiers.

The movement for legalized euthanasia, far from helping us achieve goals of that kind, actually rests upon precisely the same assumption about human need, health, and the role of medicine that have created our present crisis—the right to, and necessity of, full control over our fate. Legally available active euthanasia would worsen, not help, that crisis. By assuming that, in the face of a failure of medicine to cure our illness or stop our dying, we should have the right to be killed, the euthanasia movement gives to the value of control over self and nature too high a place at too high a social cost. The contemporary medical enterprise has increasingly become one that considers the triumph of illness and the persistence of death both a human failure and a supreme challenge still to be overcome. It is an enterprise that feeds on hope, that constantly tells itself how much farther it has to go, that takes all progress to date as simply a prologue to the further progress that can be achieved. Nothing less than total control of human nature, the banishment of its illnesses and diseases, seems to be the implicit ultimate goal.

The argument for euthanasia seems to be agreeing about the centrality and validity of control as a goal: if medicine cannot now give us the health and continued life we want, it can and should at least give us a total control over the timing and circumstances of our death, bringing its skills to bear to achieve that end. By making a denial of the distinction between killing and allowing to die central to its argument, the euthanasia movement has embodied the assumption, the conceit actually, that man is now wholly in control of everything, responsible for all life and all death. Allowing a disease to take its course is no longer to be morally distinguished from outright killing. Either way, it is our doing.

There is a clear consequence of this view: our slavery to our power over nature is now complete. Euthanasia is, in that respect, the other side of the coin of unlimited medical progress.

The compassion it seeks is not just in response to pain and suffering. It is more deeply a response to our failure to achieve final control over our destiny. That is why we cannot be rid of the pain.

The compassion is misplaced. It seems to be a way of saying that just as we have a full right to control our living, we should have a full right to control our dying. Even more, the right to control our death offers a saving antidote to our failure to control life; it makes up for the progress medicine has not yet achieved. We design a healthcare system oriented to meeting individual curative needs and then, with euthanasia, guarantee that, when the skills and knowledge of the system fail, medicine can at least give us a decisive control over our dying. The last word, long sought, becomes ours.

Yet this tactic for dealing with the failures of medicine, the inadequacies of progress, must itself fail, no less so than the system that generates it as a popular demand in response to those failures. The very drive for control, for ultimate mastery over our fate, itself generates a sense of loss and suffering when that drive fails, as it must. We have been seduced by the idea of ceaseless progress into hoping for, into insistently demanding, even better health and forestalled death. When we do not get it, we want at least (as a consolation prize) the kind of ultimate control that is the animating power behind it. This is a vicious cycle. The more power over our nature we get, the more we want; correspondingly, the more we fail to get, the more we feel its absence. If we continue to seek with our present obsessiveness ever better health, that is, ever more control over our bodily fate, we can be certain of ever greater despair when we fail to achieve it—and thus be no less certain of a rising demand for euthanasia to respond to this despair. Can we not understand how odd, how literally bizarre it is, that the greater the success of medicine in improving life and extending health, the greater the fear of illness and death and the greater the fear that the same medicine will oppress us in our dying? To turn to euthanasia as a way out of that cycle is to pour more fuel on a fire already raging out of control.

Our deepest need is just the opposite. We need to learn better how to live with our inability to bring nature under our control, how to make the most of a human condition we cannot vanquish, only ameliorate. Legalized euthanasia would be a powerful counterincentive to devise better systems of care and caring. Why should we bother if people can just do away with themselves, effectively and economically? The very premise of a philosophy of caring is that it is not necessary for human well-being always to control nature, that it is valuable to embrace the needs of those for whom medicine can do no further good—for it will always be the case that at some point medicine must fail. To give a priority to caring is to compensate for that fact and, even more, to say that the healthcare system should be something other than one dedicated to cure and control. Unbounded medical progress and euthanasia both represent efforts to ultimately triumph over our human limitations. Not only will and must that drive fail, but it most debases and suffocates the one thing we always need in the face of those limitations: to be cared for.

Yet that mistake might be nothing more than serious folly were it the only issue at stake. There is an even worse prospect. The movement to legalize euthanasia promises to corrupt our relationships with each other in the most fundamental way. It would inaugurate a move to a society that sanctions private killings and which would, moreover, make physicians the agents of this change. In their best moments, most societies have worked hard to reduce the occasions of killing. They have worked against war and against social violence and, in opposition to private moralities of oppression or vengeance, have reserved to the state the right to take life, and then only for the most pressing reasons of the public interest. When societies have failed in this effort, as they grossly and regularly have, it is usually because some individuals, or some group or other, believe that they have good reasons to kill others, usually noble reasons. Terrorism, assassinations, and killing squads are prime examples of that in our day. It may seem unfair to compare the legally sanctioned killing of patients by their doctors with that kind of lawless abuse. But the reason it has been understood as an abuse is because it moves killing from the public to the private realm; and that is a consummately dangerous move to make.

The compassion that is supposed to be served by allowing doctors to kill those patients who request it, or to help them kill themselves, is not a sufficient reason to overcome the general prohibition against private killings. To put doctors in charge of the killing, those whose profession has been most dedicated to the protection of life, is to compound the error. The private killing is to be done by those publicly charged and sanctioned to help us deal with the threat of death. Only if we think that it is the obligation of the physician to control death if he or she cannot control illness can that be a morally plausible role.

## CONTROLLING DEATH, ALLOWING DEATH

Behind the present drive to legalize euthanasia lies, then, an important consequence of a tacit belief of contemporary medicine, one well conveyed to the general public. It is the belief that medicine both can and should bring an almost ultimate control to disease and death, and that a failure to pursue all avenues that would make that possible should be understood as a culpable failure. It is an attitude that lies in part behind the malpractice problem as well, the fruit of too high patient expectations of physician perfection. Increasingly, a failure of Congress to appropriate sufficient money for biomedical research is treated as a moral dereliction—if disease might be cured, we ought to try to cure it; it is wrong not to make the effort.

A very similar kind of belief has thoroughly bedeviled efforts to terminate treatment on dying patients, or on those for whom further treatment will bring no benefit. For if ultimate control is believed to be the appropriate goal, the relinquishment of control—allowing a disease to take its course and a person to die—must necessarily be seen as a failure. A strong enough effort was not made. This is precisely what physicians report about their own attitudes toward dying patients for whom they can do nothing more. They feel guilty, as if they have personally let the patient, and the patient's family, down. The agenda of the National Institutes of Health supports this interpretation. By pursuing all known causes of disease, death, and disability, it expresses its faith that they are amenable to ultimate control, and that it is appropriate to seek such control, indeed wrong not to seek it. It treats all known causes of death, moreover, as evils. It did not, to be sure, invent that kind of stance. It is one that is supported, and believed, by the society as a whole. It is one of our most powerful national myths.

If an ideology of control lies behind the euthanasia movement, it is powerfully abetted by the fear that people have of death in the hands of contemporary medicine. For a growing number of people, almost anything looks better than having one's life saved and extended by that very medicine meant to improve it. There is likely to be only one effective remedy for this situation. Patients must have a strong assurance that they will, if they want, and if it is appropriate, be allowed to die. That means altering the reigning ideology of aggressive treatment that lies behind the medical care they will receive and those predispositions and practices that lead to what is widely perceived as excessive treatment. At the least, this will require a solution to the malpractice crisis, a source of unnecessary treatment. No less will it require more effective means of palliation—particularly drugs to relieve pain—and a greater willingness to use them. Above all, it will be necessary to demonstrate, by word and deed, that patients need not fear excessive, unwanted treatment, precisely the fear that stimulates a desire for active euthanasia. It is here that a failure to give sufficient weight to caring—sacrificed in a dedication to curing—comes to have a profoundly harmful result. Patients come to believe that they are, or will be, in the hands of a system that must *do* something to them and with them, that it must intervene not to care and comfort but to change outcomes and dominate nature. A good intention, to cure, gets out of hand and the main purpose, the patient's welfare, is lost.

I write those words with a great sense of trepidation. There is, on the one hand, the danger of seeming to suggest that all treatment of the dying is inappropriate and unwanted, and that is clearly false, or of seeming to suggest that nothing of value is now being done to deal with that problem, which is no less clearly false. There is, on the other hand, the danger of going too far, of allowing to die those who should have a chance, and a right, to live on. I have suggested that one reason it is so difficult to terminate treatment, even when almost everyone wants and can justify it, is that the contemporary drive to treat displays the confluence of two powerful currents: a cultural respect for individual life, and a medical commitment to preserving life. One should be exceedingly careful in tampering with either of them. Yet some alterations are necessary. We need to understand that a respect for individual life does not entail an unlimited effort to employ at whatever cost every technological possibility to preserve that life, and that it is a wrong view of medicine that it should seek to bring total control over life and death and be judged a failure when it does not do so. Those attitudes, never a part of the historical tradition of medical ethics, have crept into medical practice; they need to be curbed.

Is there a practical point of leverage where a shift of this kind might be expressed, and could that be done without the introduction of great moral hazards? There is such a point. It is to modify the now-standard presumption that, when in doubt with critically ill patients, it is better to treat than not treat, to act rather than not act. That presumption—which has from all evidence become stronger in parallel with medicine's increased efficacy—loses its otherwise good moral sense when technology can almost always extend life for some additional time, however poor its condition. That is because medicine can preserve organs or organ function far better than it can preserve the entire person whose organs they are. That is medicine's peculiar and disturbing power as death draws near, and attention is thereby distracted from the impending death of that person, hidden by the technological intervention.

We must find a way to change that situation, and that could be done by modifying the presumption always to treat and to act.

That modification should take the form of a great reluctance to use curative, life-extending technology in the care of the critically ill, likely terminal, or irreversibly declining patient, unless two conditions are simultaneously met. The first is that there would have to be a *good* probability that it will *significantly* modify the course of the underlying illness, by arresting or reversing its advance, and the second is that the long-term outcome for the patient as a person promises to be a good one. I will call that the *benefit presumption test*, meaning to suggest that to use a technology there should be a positive presumption that the patient will benefit.

The goal here is to let the patient's condition and the long-term prognosis (not the mere forestalling of death) determine whether to make use of those technologies that can artificially sustain the body. The test is what a technology will do for the overall life and welfare of a patient, not what it will do to forestall a coming death or to sustain organ systems. A cardiopulmonary resuscitation (CPR) in the case of an advanced terminally ill cancer patient, the introduction of an artificial feeding tube for a patient who there is good reason to believe has lapsed into permanent vegetative state, and intensive neonatal efforts with a low-birthweight, seriously harmed infant provide examples of cases where an application of the "benefit presumption test" would be appropriate. In cases where severe budgetary limits are required, the benefit presumption test could be formulated into categorical standards, establishing a uniform test to be applied to all patients. The point is to retain respect for the value of individual human life, the dignity of the life, while not becoming slaves to our available technology, exactly what now seems to have happened.

We must, in short, work to change the cultural context in which the care of patients takes place, and that means changing those fundamental perspectives that bespeak more the ambition and hubris of technological medicine and its drive to control nature than a reflection of human ends and experience carefully considered. The means of medicine have come to dominate the proper ends of medicine. The ends of medicine have never entailed the necessity to banish illness and death or demand full control over our finite biological nature.

Institutionally, this would mean putting in place a number of procedures and guidelines that would make it easier to terminate treatment, to reverse the present force of technology. They include protocols to carefully control admission to critical-care medicine in the first place, guidelines for the termination of treatment, and legal protection of families and physicians who make decisions to terminate treatment. There are many such valuable protocols and guidelines already available and I will not lay out here the various means that might be employed.[23] The main and most difficult problem does not, in any event, lie in those details. They have been polished and elaborated for well over two decades in this country with far less success and impact than they deserve. Why is that? Because they have to cope with the overwhelming bias to treat, to keep going. The burden of proof remains on those who want to stop, much too heavily so.

That burden of proof will have to be modified.[24] If we come to accept the ideas that medicine neither can nor should try to meet all individual curative needs; that efficiency does not offer us a way out; that government has a right to look to societal and not individual benefits in its support of curative medicine; that people need care more than cure; that a longer life is not necessarily a happier life; that technology can bewitch us to provide curative efforts that do the patient, as patient, no good; that medicine falsifies its role when it seeks ultimate control of life and death—if we accepted all that, we would already have gone a long way toward shifting the burden of proof. We would have introduced a number of balancing considerations to dampen the hubris of a one-dimensional technological medicine—always prone by its nature to be used because it does something, providing a kind of comforting reassurance—and thus to make it serve our ends rather than its ends. One of our human ends, not unimportant, is to be allowed to die when nothing more of any serious value can be done for us.

# CHAPTER 9

# MODERNIZING MORTALITY: MEDICAL PROGRESS AND THE GOOD SOCIETY

In Condorcet's history of human progress, published in 1795, he wrote the memorable words that to this day animate the enterprise of scientific medicine: "Would it be absurd then to suppose that this perfection of the human species might be capable of indefinite progress; that the day will come when death will only be due only to extraordinary accidents or to the decay of the vital forces, and that ultimately, the average span between birth and decay will have no assignable value? Certainly man will not become immortal, but will not the interval between the first breath that he draws and the time when in the natural course of events, without disease or accident, he expires, increase indefinitely?"[1]

Such optimism is rarely expressed so unguardedly any longer; we have become more restrained than the French *philosophes*. Yet the enthusiasm with which the possibilities of medical research are advanced in Congress and elsewhere, the hopes that are held out by medical scientists for the conquest of every known disease, and the public commitment to medical advancement show how deeply embedded is its power. At regular intervals, the old optimism surfaces, as when Lewis Thomas once said that he expected most major diseases of the present to be as well understood as the infectious diseases of the past, or when the present Director General of the World Health Organization, Dr. Hiroshi Nakajima, stated that "the right to a long life, which might theoretically be averaged at 100 years, is a basic human right of every individual."[2]

The tragedy and complexity of our present situation are not that such prophecies and optimism have been proved false, thus abandoning us to our present bodily fates. Medical and scientific advances continue to come at a fast pace, and each one seems to open the way for still another. We do not yet know how long average life expectancy might be, or whether we can rid ourselves of most of our present diseases and infirmities. Those who have predicted the failure of this or that scientific dream have probably been more wrong over time than those who predicted their success. I do not, then, want to make a brief against the possibility of further medical progress, even Condorect's "indefinite progress." He has yet to be proved false, even if we can debate whether every medical advance should be called progress

That point, however, is neither the end of the story nor the whole story. Only now have we come to see with any clarity the individual and social results of desiring, and trying to pay for, that kind of progress. We have found our mortality wanting, and we have tried to modernize it. What have we learned? At the least we know that it can be an extraordinarily expensive economic venture, consuming resources at a rapid and growing rate, in lock step with the progress. Save perhaps in the care of the dying, we have been less slow to notice, or concede, the high human costs of chasing that progress. We have been reluctant to note, for instance, that one reason we come to want indefinite progress is that we constantly upgrade our needs to stay one jump ahead of our achievements; the more we get, the more we want. We manage to keep ourselves dissatisfied, no matter how much better off we become. This is an old story in human affairs. We have added something new to it, however. There is the fear of aging and death in the company of modern medicine; the greater sense of illness and vulnerability that the progress ironically instills in us; the growing inability to find a way of coming to grips with the reality of death, a reality now seemingly transformed into wrenching choice rather than a deliverance of fate; and the anxiety occasioned by our capacity to transform our biological condition without a comparable capacity to transform our social condition.

That was not supposed to happen. We were meant to overcome obstacles, to transform our human fate. We do not know what to do when we fail, as we must. As Michael Ignatieff has observed, "The modern world, for very good reasons, does not have a vernacular of fate. Cultures that live by the values of self-realization and self-mastery are not especially good at dying, at submitting to those experiences where freedom ends and biological fate begins. Why should they be? Their strong side is Promethean ambition: the defiance and transcendence of fate, material, and social limit. Their weak side is submitting to the inevitable."[3] In our allocation of healthcare resources, we have an additional jeopardy. We have been able neither to overcome our biological fate nor to wisely manage the resources necessary to accommodate even that fate we have mastered.

René Dubos once wrote movingly of the "mirage of health." "Complete and lasting freedom from disease," he observed, "is but a dream remembered from imaginings of a Garden of Eden."[4] We have yet to enfold within our modern thinking about healthcare the implications of that simple, but profound truth. If we cannot conquer all disease, or avoid all accidents, or overcome aging and death—*not now, not ever*—what should that truth mean for the devising of a healthcare system?

## GOOD HEALTH AND THE GOOD SOCIETY

We can begin responding to that question by changing our understanding of medical progress, especially that version which seeks "indefinite progress." If that is construed to mean the meeting of all individual need for cure and the avoidance of death, it is a hopeless and ultimately damaging quest. If it might, instead, be understood as an effort to determine how best to live within the boundaries of a finite body and finite resources, then our task becomes one of finding a good balance and equilibrium, and of aiming for the kind of progress that most promotes it. I have tried to capture some of that idea with the image of implosion rather than explosion as a goal for the system. It would be an intensification inward—improving, so to speak, the interior of a modest, affordable room rather than aspiring to always enlarge the room, and that room itself set within a human dwelling whose ensemble of rooms is well proportioned and coherent.

How could a goal of this kind be made plausible? The obstacles are powerful. "What has happened in the modern world," Michael Walzer has noted, "is simply that disease itself, even when it is endemic rather than epidemic, has come to be seen as a plague. And since the plague can be dealt with, it *must* be dealt with. People will not endure what they no longer believe they have to endure."[5] Yet we must persuade people—persuade those people who are *ourselves*—that we will have to endure illness and death, convince ourselves that we are wrong in thinking we no longer have to endure disease. We will have to be convinced that a single-minded ambition to overcome mortality will generate individual misery and societal distortion, that it will create a house, our society, in which we would not want to live. We will have to be persuaded that our desire for progress, understandable enough, can be preserved but now pointed in a different direction, one designed to enrich and intensify, not to enlarge and conquer.

Consider what we now do in providing healthcare. We focus on individual medical needs and wants, devise graphs of death and illness, work up biomedical research lists, and then seek as much money as can be had—and no amount is too much—to meet those demands. Not surprisingly, they are insistent demands, mainly because they involve all of us, if not now then tomorrow, and because they touch on our life and our death, a subject that tends to capture our attention. As a consequence, we make health an obsession and then try to spend our way out of it, and the cure soon becomes its own kind of disease. The result is clearly seen in the growing proportion of the GNP going to health. It muscles aside everything else.

The corrective cannot come from within the domain of health, which has no intrinsic limits. It can only come from a coherent perspective on the general welfare of the society as a whole and of the individuals who compose it. That perspective is the only shield against those unending lists of statistics to show how many workdays are lost from illness, or how many diseases are yet to be cured, or how many individual needs are going unmet, or how many wondrous research possibilities there are. Their irresistible force must be met by one just as powerful. That can only be the force of understanding that the welfare of our social, educational, economic, and cultural institutions—and the happiness of the individuals who draw their sustenance from those institutions—must be well nourished if health is to have a point and a context. For it is their flourishing which is the point of good health. If health becomes an end in itself, then its quest begins to craze and impoverish us. That is all we will have, and we cannot forever hang on to that anyway.

The best medicine for a good society is that which contributes to the health necessary to make the society function well, to achieve its appropriate ends. The measure of that achievement is twofold: the sufficiency of general health to assure the viability of its social, cultural, and political institutions; and its willingness to guarantee to its citizens a decent baseline of public health and individual caring, and then beyond that as much—and only as much—individualized cure as is compatible with overall societal needs. The best society for a good medicine is one which understands that it has many needs and many dimensions, of which health is only one and itself a means to other ends rather than an end in itself. It will be a society which comprehends that, however understandable and insistent the individual desire to overcome illness and forestall death, it must at some point be resisted in order that other human ends can be sought and nourished, those that together respond to the full range of individual and social possibilities. A society excessively bent on conquering illness and death is certain both to fail and to harm many other values and human goods in the process. Life is to be lived for the sake of living a life, not for the sake of avoiding death.

The misery of disease and the hope for cure are powerful motivations. It will thus not be an easy task to shift our priorities to a different kind of medical progress, and to a more rounded, modest conception of the place of health in our individual destinies and in our common life together. Such a shift can only be built upon a public discussion and debate of a kind heavily resisted in this country, and it would require a consensus of a kind many would consider dangerous. We will have to talk together about what kind and level of health is sufficient for the good functioning of society; and that will mean trying to devise together a picture of a coherent, well-proportioned society, one that finds a valid mix of health, education, defense, housing, welfare, culture, and recreation. We should, as Herbert Stein has proposed, use the national budget as a way of thinking about the kind of society we want. We will no less have to talk together about the place of health in our individual lives. What is it reasonable to aspire to, what health *ought* we to want (as distinguished from what we do want), what lack of health can we with help endure and learn to accept? We will have to talk about the kinds of demands it is reasonable to make upon our neighbor, our tax-paying fellow citizens, for care and for cure if we are unable to afford it ourselves. What do we owe each other, and what kind of healthcare financing system are we willing to accept to make certain we discharge those obligations? We will have, in sum, to talk about the relationship between good health and the good self, between good health and the good society.

Those are basic moral issues, and they cannot be confronted adequately without a willingness to think together about human nature and human life, and to explore as a society the old and, for many, dangerously troubling idea of the human good. Yet if that idea is troubling, a shock to the notion of a pluralistic society that neither invokes nor shares a common view of the good, it is no less troubling to ignore it. The need to allocate resources among many societal needs, and to ration curative medicine within the sphere of healthcare, requires some degree of satisfying consensus. Simply to limit healthcare is not enough. That can be done brutally, by the force of political coercion. A humane consensus to limit healthcare requires a meaningful rationale, a way of looking at society and individual life as a whole, that makes some sense to those who will have to accept the limits. The more we can agree on the kind of society we want, and the sensible place of healthcare within it, the more likely we are to accept those limits. They will be our own self-imposed limits, a part of some full vision of the good of people and society.

We will in the future have to pay an increasingly large share of our healthcare costs out of our own pockets. Almost all of the various healthcare proposals now being discussed have that as their message, either explicitly or implicitly. We will have to make choices about the kind of coverage we want, and what we are willing to help pay for and what we are willing to forgo. Even a good program of guaranteed universal care for the indigent will not obviate that trend for everyone else. The consequence is that we will have to give much more thought to the place of health in our private lives. How much of it can we afford to pay for? How much *ought* we be willing to spend of our own money? To ask that question will be to ask how much we should value freedom from the threat of illness, from the danger of death. It will make us ask what kinds of lives we want to live, and how the quest for health should fit into that life.

We can, of course, ask such questions wholly in private, but we would be much better advised to talk about them together, to hear what others have to say and how others have chosen to live. We will need each other's help. Since our decisions to spend money on health will affect the lives of others, there will be some serious moral questions to consider. How much risk of poor or impaired health should young parents run? Do the elderly have an obligation to avoid burdening their children with health or long-term care costs? That question will probably once again surface as the elderly are forced to pay a larger share of their healthcare costs. Or is it the other way around, that children have an obligation to take up the financial burdens of parental care—and, if so, to what extent and in what way? To think about questions of that kind will require our mutual help and enlightenment. They are all questions about the human good. We can pretend, or insist, that they are out of place in a free, pluralistic society, one that allows each individual to invent or discover his or her own human good. But that is a form of self-deception. They are real questions, and the kind we cannot well answer entirely on our own. Nor are they necessarily proof against the discovery of a consensus, a common way of looking at things, which we will find helpful and satisfactory, even if not perfect.

We have generally failed, both experts and laypeople, to understand the way in which changing ideas of health bring with them changing ideas of our way of life and how, in turn, changes in our way of life work back into alterations of our notions of health. To understand that is already to recognize that the supposed private sphere of our individual notions of health and happiness is deeply influenced by the society in which we live. It provides us with our images, stories, and paradigms. To grasp the way our public and private ideas of health work on and with each other is thus vital. It is undeniably a puzzle of uncertain dimensions, but at the core of the problem that faces us.

If, for instance, we believe that all pain and suffering ought to be eradicated, whatever the cost to other goods and values, we will have no alternative but to give the highest priority to healthcare. If, moreover, we also believe that health and a sense of well-being are private and uniquely personal matters, then we are likely as a society to resist any common judgment about their meaning and value. We will favor policies of maximum individual choice. But it is precisely policies based on those values that are collapsing, because they have become too expensive to implement and have produced too little individual satisfaction. "What Americans need," Michael Ignatieff has written, "is a little bit of irony, a capacity to see that they are making themselves ill with the frantic pursuit of health."[6]

All of this is to say that we will have to talk openly and

forthrightly about what is actually good for us, individually and societally, and we will need some agreement, some workable shared view on what it is. We can continue talking about the problem in the acceptable language of politics and economics, of interests and trade-offs, trying to balance and adjudicate individual wants and preferences. But we should know that it is precisely that approach which has brought us deep trouble. Neither a coherent society nor a coherent healthcare system can be fashioned out of a mixture of demands that is prepared to let the clamor for improved health dominate other societal needs, that seeks unbounded medical progress, and that champions the right of individuals to define their health and other needs as they see fit.

The inevitable result in our political system is a debate carried on in the language of money, a necessary but limited language to decently encompass all the moral and social values at stake in healthcare. What can be the meaning of the familiar language, say, of "trade-offs" as a way of resolving struggles about the provision of healthcare? Lacking any common ideas of individual good save that of self-determination and self-definition, it is a recipe for the play of power and interests, winner take all, not a reflection of what might be best for people. What can it mean to talk about freedom of choice if that freedom becomes a war of all against all, each seeking maximum benefits maximally defined? That is a prescription for the ruination of all. What can it mean to seek "indefinite progress" in health if the cost of seeking it is to impoverish the rest of our lives?

Can we talk about "what is best for people," with all the overtones of moral judgment and substantive consensus that a phrase like that conveys? My response is: How can we not, finally, come to talk about that? Will we not in any event be talking about it implicitly, even if we try to stifle it? We already think that, in some sense, health is important. That is itself one facet of a view of the human good; a general stance has been taken. Now the task is to discover how, and in what way, health is important. There is no wholly neutral standpoint from which to do that. Since we must, moreover, come to some common political judgment about the allocation of healthcare resources, we will have to find a way to put together in some coherent fashion our various views on health and human life. We cannot solve our problem otherwise, except meanly and poorly, and we cannot avoid tacit and concealed answers to questions about the human good no matter what kind of solution we adopt.

Nor need we despair in advance of getting somewhere. We have much of value with which we can work, in our experience as well as our traditions. We have had at least fifty years of experience with high-technology medicine, and we should have learned something by now. The most important insight is the most simple: it is just like everything else in the world. It can bring good and it can bring harm, and often at the same time. It bewitches us as much as it benefits us. In the company of this technology, we have had the experience in the United States of seeing how the demand for healthcare increases the more of it we get, but also how other cultures respond variously to that demand, and how different kinds of healthcare systems can be devised to cope with it. We have had the experience of discovering, if we look, that the connection between health and happiness remains both important and yet indeterminate; there is no perfect symmetry. More research, of the right kind, could well improve that symmetry, but simply throwing one new device or drug after another at illness is not necessarily the way to go about it. If nothing else, our experience should have tutored us to understand that changes in the way we live our lives, the way we relate to our environment, can make the greatest difference of all to our good health. Of course, that is something we have known for a long time, but it sometimes seems to require hard experience to recall what we have always known.

## EFFICIENCY AND MORTALITY

We are at an important historical juncture. Our hopes that we could avoid a genuinely serious crisis, through cost containment or other tactics, have come to all too little. That failure invites us to reconsider in a fundamental way just what it is that we should be seeking. We need to look as hard at our ends as at our means. We can reject that invitation and run away from the harsh questions it will force us to consider. We can, instead, interpret our problems with cost containment, with unmet and growing needs, and with pressures to ration as simply failures of will and ingenuity, motivation and management. We can assume we have just not well learned how to make sensible trade-offs and put proper incentives in place. Cost containment has not failed; it has just never been properly tried, we can say. We can, that is, convince ourselves that the problems we have encountered in the project of modernizing mortality, in seeking indefinite progress, in hoping for more life and a better life, are just bureaucratic and organizational in nature. There is nothing wrong with the goals. We just need to seek them more efficiently.

Or we can understand those problems as evidence that there is something flawed about the project itself, about its very ends and purposes. Instead of assuming that more ingenuity and better cost-containment incentives will let us proceed apace, we might wonder whether our failures in efficiency bespeak a deeper lack of understanding of our own nature and limitations. We might wonder whether our lack of success in meeting individual health needs (always being redefined), in being able to formulate what a "decent minimum" of healthcare would encompass, is just chance or, perhaps, the beginning of insight into the hopelessness of the quest. We might wonder whether our ultimate problems with healthcare are not moral rather than practical, more about our chosen ends than our managerial means.

We have for many years now just drifted along, creating a healthcare system that not only costs too much for what it delivers, but fails to deliver what it could for millions of people. It has also drifted into some serious imbalances in what it actually brings people. It has led us to spend too much on health in comparison with other social needs, too much on the old in comparison with the young, too much on the acutely ill in comparison with the chronically ill, too much on curing in comparison with caring, too much on expensive individual health needs in comparison with less expensive societal health needs, and too much on extending the length of life rather than enhancing the quality of life.

Those are contentious convictions, but I think positions of that kind—however they may differ in detail and emphasis—will begin to emerge if we open up in a full way the moral questions. Once we have done so, we will find that they must be grappled with as moral questions. They cannot be adequately confronted if translated into more tractable political or economic problems. The relative priority we should accord the young and the old in the healthcare system, or length of life versus quality of life, or cure versus care, for example, are philosophical issues, and they need answers on their merits, however awkward politically. This will happen only if we refuse to allow ourselves to be any longer comforted by those who would put aside such questions to pursue, once again, a new try at efficiency.

Robert G. Evans, as effectively as anyone, has argued that any talk of the "inevitability of rationing" or of "painful prescriptions" simply distracts our attention from the possibilities for greater efficiency, and that we should simply get on with that task, one which is, in any event, "enough of a challenge for one generation; who knows what the next generation's technology may bring?"[7] That way of thinking has had its turn, and more than once reached its limits. We still need efficiency, but it is no longer enough, nor is it wise to limit our perspective to the present generation. Efficiency in healthcare has failed in the United States because it must fail here. Our values and institutions work against it, as Evans himself has reminded us.

Worse still, even if they did not, that would at most postpone the time of crisis. The dynamic of an aging society, technological progress, and the public appetite for improved health work against any and all inherent limits. The Canadian system that Professor Evans holds up for our admiration is itself beginning to show strains similar to ours. It will have its turn at crisis, and probably sooner rather than later.[8] As Rudolf Klein has observed of the British National Health Service: "Even if policies of prevention and social engineering were to be successfully introduced, their very success in extending life expectancy would create new demands for alleviating the chronic degenerative diseases of old age . . . no policy can ensure that people will drop dead painlessly at the age of 80, not having troubled the health services previously."[9]

The faith in economic salvation from problems of that kind should be put aside, along with the myth that a still larger research investment will allow us to turn some corner on costly care, or that a more informed, cost-conscious patient will make the decisive difference, or that technology assessment will do the trick. They are all ways of evading not just the hard choices, but the hard questions, and all the more seductive because some of them are truly needed and respond to part of the problem. But it is as if the optimism of the scientific enterprise has infected the way we think about the social enterprise, that if we can make limitless medical progress, we must therefore be able to make limitless progress in coping with its individual, economic, and social problems and costs. That is a profound mistake, but one whose power animates each new cost-containment and efficiency scheme. What will it take to convince ourselves otherwise? Still greater deterioration in our system? One more failed cost-containment plan? One more stab at improved competition? And when they fail, will we continue to berate ourselves that we have not tried hard enough? Or blame the doctors for charging too much, the juries for awarding too heavy malpractice damages, or the medical manufacturers for their cupidity? Will we, that is, round up the usual suspects?

Nothing I have said here should be taken to imply that we will not need an open political process, a policy compromise, or an adjudication of competing interests. We will never find total agreement on something as central, as constantly changing, as complex, as health and healthcare. But we need some significant degree of consensus, much more than we now have, and on matters of basic values and perspectives. The change must come from the inside, from ourselves, those selves that must wrestle with the fact that we are both patients (or would-be patients), hurting and needy, alone with our individual needs, and yet members also of local communities, families, and a larger society, whose collective well-being gives our individuality a place and an enhanced meaning. We need to search for the right fit, the right balance. To achieve that we need a new dimension to our political debates. We must not hesitate to talk about human ends and the human good, and have the nerve to let the insights that emerge enrich and guide our political struggle. We have one extraordinary advantage over our predecessors. We are the healthiest people in the history of the human race, the most medically fit to have such a struggle.

A healthcare system that took its point of departure from our need as individuals to be cared for, that promised never to abandon us, would bring us back into continuity with the richest and deepest traditions of medicine. A system that focused its research efforts on enhancing the quality of life rather than on holding off death, or on means of preventing illness and reducing the debilities of old age rather than on high-technology cures, or on enhancing the general level of public health rather than on the special curative needs of individuals, would be a more rounded and coherent system. A healthcare system which understood that it was meant to be part of, and to serve the needs of, a broader social and political system would be one less prone to think only of its own needs, or to forget that health is only a means to the living of a life, not its goal. A system that guaranteed a minimally decent level of healthcare for all, in turn asking each of us to rein in our private demands, would be a decent and manageable one. That is not an impossible ideal.

# APPENDIX: *SELECTED HEALTHCARE DATA*

The purpose of this appendix is to present some selected data, designed to illustrate themes that I have pursued in the book. The available information on health and healthcare is enormous, and all of us who study it must be selective in using it, and no less selective in determining whether, and in what ways, it supports our observations and reflections. We all hope, and perhaps secretly suspect, that the way the world really is, the true facts, will confirm our convictions. That is not always the case, and some wariness is always in order. The information provided by the tables and figures that follow is meant to be suggestive, not conclusive, about the nature of our problems and about the kind of future we are likely to face.

How serious is the economic problem of healthcare likely to be in the future? A premise of my argument is that it will be very serious, far more than can be coped with by greater efficiency alone. Table 1 presents some basic cost projections, prepared by the federal government, through to the year 2000. In 1989, we spent about $550 billion for healthcare. The projection is that, within the next eleven years, that could triple, to $1.5 trillion, and 15 percent of the GNP.

How do our expenditures compare with those of other countries? The information provided in Table 2 provides an answer to that question—we spend more, much more, than others. What difference has our spending made? The paradox of modern medical progress is nowhere more apparent than in Tables 3 and 4. Table 3 shows that there has been a significant *decline* in death rates in recent decades. Table 4, however, indicates that the decline in death rates has been accompanied by a no less significant *increase* in chronic conditions serious enough to limit activity. Those tables are also worth contemplating in the context of the discussion of the concept of a "compression of morbidity" discussed in Chapter 7.

What are the factors that account for the great increase in health-care costs? Figure 1 distinguishes among general inflation, medical-care inflation, population changes, and other factors. Among those "other factors"—35 percent in 1986—are population aging, increased individual consumption, and intensified use of technology, items of great importance in thinking about the forces and values driving our healthcare system.

Is it possible, or likely, that a greater investment in biomedical research could help us to control or bring down the costs of health-care? There are some who strongly push that view. Figure 2, published by the National Institutes of Health, unfortunately shows that there is an almost perfect correlation between the cost of healthcare and the money invested in basic research and development. To show a correlation is not, to be sure, to prove causality, but it does suggest that spending more money on research does not bring healthcare costs down. Should we expect a great change in the future? No evidence has been brought forward to support that hope.

The hope for a breakthrough in research is nowhere more powerful than in trying to meet the health needs of the elderly. What are some projections about healthcare costs for the elderly in the years ahead? I have contended that the combination of a growing number of elderly and a greater application of services and technology to the cure of the elderly will in itself create a massive problem in the years ahead. Table 5 presents the result of one important study, projecting annual deficits in the Medicare program in the range of hundreds of billions of dollars. It should be noted, moreover, that those projections are for the present Medicare system, devoted to acute-care medicine for the elderly. The figures do not include any projections for increased nursing-home costs or home-care costs for the elderly. Table 6 presents some figures about nursing-home care, however, well worth thinking about, especially in conjunction with the Medicare projections. They suggest not only that we will have to set limits on Medicare expenditures simply to keep that program under some semblance of control, but that it will be necessary to do so to make room for the long-term care needs that will have to be met.

The daunting magnitude of the task facing us in the years ahead in providing healthcare for the elderly is underscored by the realization that there will be comparatively fewer younger people to help provide such support. Table 7 provides some projections about the change in relative size of different age groups. At the same time as we are worrying about that problem, we will also have to be working to improve the health status of the poor. Figure 3 shows the result of one careful study of the correlation between socioeconomic status and sheer survival: poverty kills, by increasing the risk of death. It also makes people sicker, which is why the poor have far more health problems in general than those more well off. And of course the more people who go into old age in poor health, the more exacerbated will be the problem of providing them with good healthcare.

**TABLE 1**

**NATIONAL HEALTH EXPENDITURES—AGGREGATE AND PER CAPITA AMOUNTS, PERCENTAGE DISTRIBUTION, AND AVERAGE ANNUAL PERCENTAGE CHANGE, BY SOURCE OF FUNDS: SELECTED CALENDAR YEARS 1965–2000**

| Item | 2000 | 1995 | 1990 | 1987 | 1986 | 1985 | 1984 | 1980 | 1970 | 1965 |
|---|---|---|---|---|---|---|---|---|---|---|
| | | | | | Amount in Billions | | | | | |
| National health expenditures | $1,529.3 | $999.1 | $647.3 | $496.6 | $458.2 | $422.6 | $391.1 | $248.1 | $75.0 | $41.9 |
| Private | 879.4 | 575.5 | 378.2 | 294.8 | 268.5 | 246.6 | 231.3 | 142.9 | 47.2 | 30.9 |
| Public | 649.9 | 423.5 | 269.0 | 201.7 | 189.7 | 176.0 | 159.7 | 105.2 | 27.8 | 11.0 |
| Federal | 498.6 | 317.7 | 195.5 | 142.7 | 134.7 | 124.5 | 111.6 | 71.0 | 17.7 | 5.5 |
| State and local | 151.3 | 105.8 | 73.6 | 59.0 | 55.0 | 51.5 | 48.1 | 34.2 | 10.1 | 5.5 |
| | | | | | Per Capita Amount | | | | | |
| National health expenditures | $5,551 | $3,739 | $2,511 | $1,973 | $1,837 | $1,710 | $1,597 | $1,054 | $349 | $205 |
| Private | 3,192 | 2,154 | 1,467 | 1,172 | 1,076 | 998 | 945 | 607 | 220 | 152 |
| Public | 2,359 | 1,585 | 1,044 | 802 | 760 | 712 | 652 | 447 | 129 | 54 |
| Federal | 1,810 | 1,189 | 758 | 567 | 540 | 504 | 456 | 302 | 82 | 27 |
| State and local | 549 | 396 | 285 | 235 | 221 | 208 | 196 | 145 | 47 | 27 |
| | | | | | Percentage Distribution | | | | | |
| National health expenditures | 100.0 | 100.0 | 100.0 | 100.0 | 100.0 | 100.0 | 100.0 | 100.0 | 100.0 | 100.0 |
| Private | 57.5 | 57.6 | 58.4 | 59.4 | 58.6 | 58.4 | 59.2 | 57.6 | 63.0 | 73.8 |
| Public | 42.5 | 42.4 | 41.6 | 40.6 | 41.4 | 41.6 | 40.8 | 42.4 | 37.0 | 26.2 |
| Federal | 32.6 | 31.8 | 30.2 | 28.7 | 29.4 | 29.5 | 28.5 | 28.6 | 23.6 | 13.2 |
| State and local | 9.9 | 10.6 | 11.4 | 11.9 | 12.0 | 12.2 | 12.3 | 13.8 | 13.5 | 13.0 |
| | | | Average Annual Percentage Change from Previous Year Shown | | | | | | | |
| U.S. population | 0.6 | 0.7 | 0.8 | 0.9 | 0.9 | 0.9 | 1.0 | 0.9 | 1.0 | — |
| Gross national product | 6.4 | 6.6 | 6.9 | 5.3 | 5.2 | 6.2 | 8.3 | 10.4 | 7.6 | — |
| National health expenditures | 8.9 | 9.1 | 9.2 | 8.4 | 8.4 | 8.1 | 12.0 | 12.7 | 12.3 | — |
| Private | 8.8 | 8.8 | 8.7 | 9.8 | 8.9 | 6.6 | 12.8 | 11.7 | 8.8 | — |
| Public | 8.9 | 9.5 | 10.1 | 6.3 | 7.8 | 10.2 | 11.0 | 14.2 | 20.4 | — |
| Federal | 9.4 | 10.2 | 11.1 | 6.0 | 8.2 | 11.5 | 12.0 | 14.9 | 26.1 | — |
| State and local | 7.4 | 7.5 | 7.6 | 7.2 | 6.8 | 7.1 | 8.9 | 13.0 | 13.1 | — |
| | | | | | Number in Millions | | | | | |
| U.S. population[a] | 275.5 | 267.2 | 257.8 | 251.6 | 249.5 | 247.2 | 244.9 | 235.3 | 214.9 | 204.1 |
| | | | | | Amount in Billions | | | | | |
| Gross national product | $10,164 | $7,467 | $5,414 | $4,433 | $4,206 | $3,998 | $3,765 | $2,732 | $1,015 | $705 |
| | | | | Percentage of Gross National Product | | | | | | |
| National health expenditures | 15.0 | 13.4 | 12.0 | 11.2 | 10.9 | 10.6 | 10.4 | 9.1 | 7.4 | 5.9 |

[a] July 1 social security area population estimates.

Note: Figures for 1986 are preliminary and those for 1987–2000 are projected.

TABLE 2

**TOTAL HEALTH EXPENDITURE AS A PERCENTAGE OF GROSS DOMESTIC PRODUCT, 1960–1986**

| | 1960 | 1965 | 1970 | 1975 | 1980 | 1983 | 1984 | 1985 | 1986 |
|---|---|---|---|---|---|---|---|---|---|
| Australia | 4.6% | 4.9% | 5.0% | 5.7% | 6.6% | 6.9% | 6.9% | 6.8% | 6.8% |
| Austria | 4.6 | 5.0 | 5.4 | 7.3 | 7.9 | 7.9 | 8.0 | 8.2 | 8.0 |
| Belgium | 3.4 | 3.9 | 4.0 | 5.8 | 6.6 | 7.2 | 7.2 | 7.2 | 7.1 |
| Canada | 5.5 | 6.1 | 7.2 | 7.3 | 7.4 | 8.6 | 8.5 | 8.4 | 8.5 |
| Denmark | 3.6 | 4.8 | 6.1 | 6.5 | 6.8 | 6.6 | 6.3 | 6.1 | 6.1 |
| Finland | 4.2 | 4.9 | 5.6 | 6.2 | 6.3 | 6.6 | 6.8 | 7.3 | 7.5 |
| France | 4.2 | 5.2 | 5.6 | 6.7 | 7.4 | 8.1 | 8.4 | 8.4 | 8.5 |
| Germany | 4.7 | 5.1 | 5.5 | 7.8 | 7.9 | 8.0 | 8.1 | 8.2 | 8.1 |
| Greece | 2.9 | 3.1 | 4.0 | 4.0 | 4.2 | 4.2 | 4.0 | 4.2 | 3.9 |
| Iceland | 5.9 | 6.0 | 8.7 | 11.1 | 6.9 | 8.2 | 7.3 | 7.8 | 7.5 |
| Ireland | 4.0 | 4.4 | 5.6 | 7.7 | 8.5 | 8.0 | 8.0 | 8.0 | 7.9 |
| Italy | 3.3 | 4.0 | 4.8 | 5.8 | 6.8 | 6.7 | 6.6 | 6.7 | 6.7 |
| Japan | 3.0 | 4.5 | 4.6 | 5.6 | 6.6 | 6.9 | 6.7 | 6.6 | 6.7 |
| Luxem-bourg | — | — | 3.8 | 5.3 | 6.1 | 6.9 | 6.6 | 6.7 | 6.9 |
| Nether-lands | 3.9 | 4.4 | 6.0 | 7.7 | 8.2 | 8.6 | 8.3 | 8.3 | 8.3 |
| New Zea-land | 4.4 | 4.5 | 5.1 | 6.4 | 7.2 | 6.3 | — | — | 6.9 |
| Norway | 3.3 | 3.9 | 5.0 | 6.7 | 6.6 | 6.8 | 6.5 | 6.4 | 6.8 |
| Portugal | — | — | — | 6.4 | 5.9 | 5.4 | 5.6 | 5.6 | 5.6 |
| Spain | 2.3 | 2.7 | 4.1 | 5.1 | 5.9 | 6.3 | 6.0 | 6.0 | 6.0 |
| Sweden | 4.7 | 5.6 | 7.2 | 8.0 | 9.5 | 9.6 | 9.5 | 9.4 | 9.1 |
| Switzer-land | 3.3 | 3.8 | 5.2 | 7.1 | 7.2 | 7.8 | 7.7 | 7.9 | 8.0 |
| Turkey | — | — | — | — | — | 3.5 | — | — | 3.6 |
| United Kingdom | 3.9 | 4.1 | 4.5 | 5.5 | 5.8 | 6.2 | 6.2 | 6.1 | 6.2 |
| United States | 5.2 | 6.0 | 7.4 | 8.4 | 9.2 | 10.7 | 10.5 | 10.7 | 11.1 |
| Mean | 4.1 | 4.6 | 5.4 | 6.7 | 7.1 | 7.2 (7.3)[a] | 7.3 | 7.3 | 7.2 (7.3)[a] |

[a] Mean excluding Turkey.

**TABLE 3**

## CHANGE IN DEATH RATES, BY AGE, UNITED STATES, 1950–1984[1]

| Age Group | (percent) | | |
|---|---|---|---|
| | **1950–1984** | **1950–1970** | **1970–1984** |
| All ages | | | |
|   Age-adjusted death rate | −35.1 | −15.1 | −23.6 |
|   Crude death rate | −10.5 | −1.9 | −8.8 |
| Under 1 | −67.1 | −35.1 | −49.3 |
| 1–4 | −62.8 | −39.4 | −38.6 |
| 5–14 | −55.6 | −31.3 | −46.6 |
| 15–24 | −24.4 | −0.3 | −24.2 |
| 25–34 | −32.2 | −11.9 | −23.1 |
| 35–44 | −42.9 | −12.3 | −35.8 |
| 45–54 | −39.0 | −14.5 | −28.6 |
| 55–64 | −32.6 | −13.2 | −22.4 |
| 65–74 | −30.0 | −11.9 | −20.5 |
| 75–84 | −31.4 | −14.2 | −20.1 |
| 85 and over | −24.6 | −13.2 | −13.2 |

TABLE 4

**PREVALENCE OF LIMITATION OF ACTIVITY
DUE TO CHRONIC CONDITIONS AND NUMBER OF CONDITIONS PER
PERSON, BY SEX AND AGE, 1969–1971 AND 1979–1981**

| Sex and Age | 1969–1971 | 1979–1981 | Percentage Change |
|---|---|---|---|
| | *Prevalence (rate per 1,000 persons)* | | |
| Total | 118.66 | 144.55 | 21.8 |
| Males | 124.43 | 146.70 | 17.9 |
| Females | 113.30 | 142.54 | 25.8 |
| Age | | | |
| Under 17 | 27.54 | 38.47 | 39.7 |
| 17–44 | 76.77 | 86.03 | 12.1 |
| 45–64 | 197.75 | 239.66 | 21.2 |
| 65–74 | 363.14 | 412.57 | 13.6 |
| 75–84 | 508.33 | 506.80 | −0.3 |
| 85 and over | 667.34 | 648.63 | −2.8 |
| | *Limiting Conditions per Person* | | |
| Total | 1.318 | 1.483 | 12.5 |
| Males | 1.306 | 1.446 | 10.7 |
| Females | 1.331 | 1.519 | 14.1 |
| Age | | | |
| Under 17 | 1.135 | 1.197 | 5.5 |
| 17–44 | 1.172 | 1.268 | 8.2 |
| 45–64 | 1.352 | 1.557 | 15.2 |
| 65–74 | 1.420 | 1.618 | 13.9 |
| 75–84 | 1.449 | 1.655 | 14.2 |
| 85 and over | 1.378 | 1.608 | 16.7 |

**TABLE 5**

## MEDICARE'S TOTAL FISCAL GAP

| | Percentage of GNP | Percentage of Payroll | Percentage of Projected Program Revenues Under Current Tax Burdens | Percentage of Projected Program Expenditures | Billions of Dollars in Relation to 1990 GNP |
|---|---|---|---|---|---|
| | | | *Intermediate Assumptions* | | |
| 1990 | 0.07 | 0.11 | 2.7 | 3.6 | 4.0 |
| 1995 | 0.34 | 0.49 | 12.2 | 14.4 | 18.3 |
| 2000 | 0.51 | 0.73 | 18.0 | 20.0 | 27.3 |
| 2005 | 0.67 | 0.95 | 23.3 | 24.6 | 35.8 |
| 2010 | 0.84 | 1.20 | 29.0 | 29.0 | 45.1 |
| 2015 | 1.09 | 1.55 | 37.0 | 34.4 | 58.4 |
| 2020 | 1.43 | 2.05 | 47.7 | 40.6 | 77.1 |
| 2025 | 1.84 | 2.63 | 59.6 | 46.4 | 99.1 |
| 2030 | 2.18 | 3.11 | 68.8 | 50.2 | 117.0 |
| 2035 | 2.36 | 3.38 | 73.8 | 52.2 | 127.2 |
| | | | *Pessimistic Assumptions* | | |
| 1990 | 0.18 | 0.26 | 6.7 | 8.4 | 9.8 |
| 1995 | 0.72 | 1.02 | 25.1 | 25.9 | 38.6 |
| 2000 | 1.16 | 1.66 | 39.4 | 35.6 | 62.5 |
| 2005 | 1.64 | 2.35 | 54.0 | 43.4 | 88.3 |
| 2010 | 2.21 | 3.16 | 70.0 | 50.2 | 118.8 |
| 2015 | 2.97 | 4.24 | 89.6 | 56.8 | 159.7 |
| 2020 | 3.92 | 5.60 | 111.7 | 62.5 | 210.9 |
| 2025 | 4.97 | 7.10 | 133.3 | 67.0 | 267.5 |
| 2030 | 5.81 | 8.30 | 148.3 | 69.7 | 312.7 |
| 2035 | 6.23 | 8.89 | 154.7 | 70.9 | 334.9 |

**TABLE 6**

**EXPENDITURES FOR NURSING-HOME CARE—AGGREGATE AND PER CAPITA AMOUNTS AND PERCENTAGE DISTRIBUTION, BY SOURCE OF FUNDS: SELECTED CALENDAR YEARS 1980–2000**

| Year | Total | Direct Patient Payments | Third Parties | | | | | | | |
| | | | All Third Parties | Private Health Insurance | Other Private Funds | Total | Government | | Medicare[a] | Medicaid[b] |
| | | | | | | | Federal | State and Local | | |
|---|---|---|---|---|---|---|---|---|---|---|
| | | | | | | *Amount in Billions* | | | | |
| 1980 | $20.4 | $8.9 | $11.5 | $0.2 | $0.1 | $11.2 | $6.0 | $5.2 | $0.4 | $9.8 |
| 1985 | 35.0 | 17.5 | 17.5 | 0.3 | 0.2 | 17.0 | 9.4 | 7.5 | 0.6 | 14.8 |
| 1986 | 38.1 | 19.4 | 18.7 | 0.3 | 0.3 | 18.1 | 10.1 | 8.0 | 0.6 | 15.8 |
| 1987 | 41.6 | 21.1 | 20.5 | 0.4 | 0.3 | 19.8 | 11.1 | 8.8 | 0.6 | 17.3 |
| 1990 | 54.5 | 28.0 | 26.6 | 0.7 | 0.4 | 25.4 | 14.3 | 11.1 | 0.8 | 22.1 |
| 1995 | 84.7 | 44.2 | 40.5 | 2.2 | 0.6 | 37.6 | 21.1 | 16.5 | 1.2 | 32.4 |
| 2000 | 129.0 | 68.5 | 60.5 | 6.2 | 1.0 | 53.3 | 29.9 | 23.4 | 1.8 | 45.0 |
| | | | | | | *Per Capita Amount* | | | | |
| 1980 | $87 | $38 | $49 | $1 | $1 | $48 | $26 | $22 | —[c] | —[c] |
| 1985 | 141 | 71 | 71 | 1 | 1 | 69 | 38 | 30 | —[c] | —[c] |
| 1986 | 153 | 78 | 75 | 1 | 1 | 73 | 41 | 32 | —[c] | —[c] |
| 1987 | 165 | 84 | 82 | 2 | 1 | 79 | 44 | 35 | —[c] | —[c] |
| 1990 | 211 | 108 | 103 | 3 | 2 | 99 | 56 | 43 | —[c] | —[c] |
| 1995 | 317 | 166 | 151 | 8 | 2 | 141 | 79 | 62 | —[c] | —[c] |
| 2000 | 468 | 248 | 220 | 23 | 4 | 193 | 108 | 85 | —[c] | —[c] |
| | | | | | | *Percentage Distribution* | | | | |
| 1980 | 100.0 | 43.6 | 56.4 | 0.9 | 0.6 | 54.9 | 29.6 | 25.3 | 1.9 | 48.0 |
| 1985 | 100.0 | 49.9 | 50.1 | 0.9 | 0.7 | 48.5 | 26.9 | 21.6 | 1.7 | 42.4 |
| 1986 | 100.0 | 51.0 | 49.0 | 0.8 | 0.7 | 47.5 | 26.6 | 20.9 | 1.6 | 41.4 |
| 1987 | 100.0 | 50.7 | 49.3 | 0.9 | 0.7 | 47.7 | 26.6 | 21.0 | 1.6 | 41.7 |
| 1990 | 100.0 | 51.3 | 48.7 | 1.3 | 0.7 | 46.7 | 26.3 | 20.4 | 1.5 | 40.6 |
| 1995 | 100.0 | 52.2 | 47.8 | 2.6 | 0.8 | 44.4 | 25.0 | 19.4 | 1.5 | 38.2 |
| 2000 | 100.0 | 53.1 | 46.9 | 4.8 | 0.8 | 41.3 | 23.2 | 18.1 | 1.4 | 34.9 |

[a] Subset of federal funds.
[b] Subset of federal and state and local funds.
[c] Calculation of per capita estimates is inappropriate.
Note: Per capita amounts based on July 1 social security area population estimates.

TABLE 7

## THE ABSOLUTE AND RELATIVE SIZES OF
## VARIOUS POPULATION GROUPS, 1965–2035

| | Population in Millions | | Aged as a Percentage of Total Population | Aged as a Percentage of Working-Age Population | Aged 80+ as a Percentage of Working-Age Population[a] |
|---|---|---|---|---|---|
| | 20–64 | 65+ | | | |
| | | *Actuals* | | | |
| 1965 | 105.0 | 19.1 | 9.4 | 18.2 | 2.9 |
| 1970 | 113.2 | 20.8 | 9.7 | 18.4 | 3.3 |
| 1975 | 122.8 | 23.3 | 10.4 | 19.0 | 3.7 |
| 1980 | 134.2 | 26.1 | 11.1 | 19.4 | 3.9 |
| 1985 | 145.1 | 28.9 | 11.7 | 19.9 | 4.2 |
| | | *Intermediate Assumptions* | | | |
| 1990 | 152.2 | 31.9 | 12.4 | 21.0 | 5.0 |
| 1995 | 158.2 | 34.3 | 12.8 | 21.7 | 5.5 |
| 2000 | 164.8 | 35.6 | 12.9 | 21.6 | 6.0 |
| 2005 | 172.0 | 37.1 | 13.1 | 21.6 | 6.6 |
| 2010 | 176.8 | 40.4 | 13.9 | 22.9 | 6.8 |
| 2015 | 177.6 | 46.2 | 15.5 | 26.0 | 6.9 |
| 2020 | 175.8 | 53.1 | 17.5 | 30.2 | 7.2 |
| 2025 | 172.1 | 60.9 | 19.7 | 35.4 | 8.3 |
| 2030 | 169.7 | 66.7 | 21.4 | 39.3 | 10.3 |
| 2035 | 170.1 | 69.0 | 22.0 | 40.6 | 12.1 |
| | | *Pessimistic Assumptions* | | | |
| 1990 | 151.8 | 32.0 | 12.5 | 21.1 | 5.1 |
| 1995 | 157.1 | 34.7 | 13.1 | 22.1 | 5.8 |
| 2000 | 163.2 | 36.4 | 13.5 | 22.3 | 6.5 |
| 2005 | 169.8 | 38.4 | 13.9 | 22.6 | 7.3 |
| 2010 | 173.7 | 42.2 | 15.1 | 24.3 | 7.9 |
| 2015 | 172.7 | 48.7 | 17.3 | 28.2 | 8.3 |
| 2020 | 168.4 | 56.4 | 19.9 | 33.5 | 9.1 |
| 2025 | 161.6 | 65.2 | 23.0 | 40.3 | 10.8 |
| 2030 | 155.3 | 72.2 | 25.6 | 46.5 | 13.7 |
| 2035 | 151.1 | 75.6 | 27.2 | 50.0 | 17.0 |

[a] Calculations of the aged 80+ are based on census projections employing demographic assumptions which are similar, though not strictly comparable, to the intermediate and pessimistic assumptions of the Social Security Trustees' report.

**FIGURE 1.** Factors affecting change in personal healthcare expenditures of billions of dollars: calendar years 1966–1986. Price inflation has always accounted for a substantial part of the increase in personal healthcare expenditures. From 1985 to 1986, 32 percent of the $33 billion increase in that spending was attributable to economywide price inflation, and another 22 percent to medical–care price inflation in excess of the general rate of price inflation. Population growth accounted for 11 percent of the change, and the remainder was attributed to other factors—changes in consumption per capita and in "intensity" as a result of rising income levels, aging of the population, and so on.

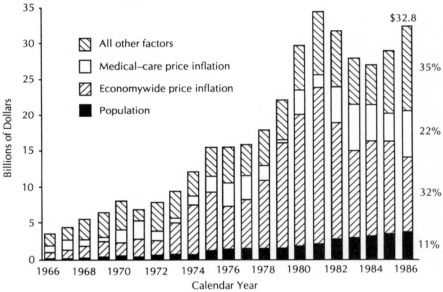

**FIGURE 2.** Percentage change since 1978 in total health costs, total R&D, and health R&D, 1979–1987.

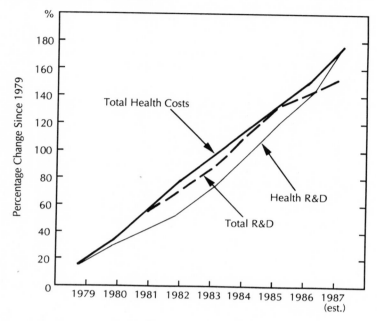

**FIGURE 3.** Health and socioeconomic status. Eighteen-year survival of Alameda County, California, residents by family income.

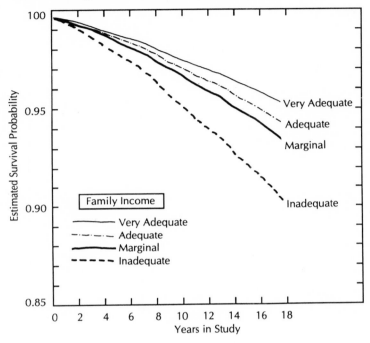

# ACKNOWLEDGMENTS

Table 1. Division of National Cost Estimates, Office of the Actuary, Health Care Financing Administration, "National Health Expenditures, 1986–2000," *Health Care Financing Review*, 8:4 (Summer 1987), p. 23.

Table 2. George J. Schieber and Jean-Pierre Poulier, "International Health Spending and Utilization Trends," *Health Affairs* (Fall 1988), p. 106, the source of which is *Measuring Health Care 1960–1983* (Paris: Organization for Economic Cooperation and Development, 1985); and updated. Reprinted with permission of *Health Affairs*.

Table 3. Dorothy Rice and Mitchell P. LaPlante, "Chronic Illness, Disability, and Increasing Longevity," in Sean Sullivan and Marion Ein Lewin, eds., *The Economics and Ethics of Long-Term Care and Disability* (Washington, D.C.: 1988), Table 2-2. Reprinted with permission of the American Enterprise Institute for Public Policy Research.

Table 4. Ibid., Table 2-8. Reprinted with permission of the American Enterprise Institute for Public Policy Research.

Table 5. John Holahan and John L. Palmer, "Medicare's Fiscal Problems: An Imperative for Reform." Reprinted with permission from *Journal of Health Politics, Policy and Law*, 13:1. Copyright © 1988 by Duke University Press.

Table 6. Division of National Cost Estimates, Office of the Actuary, Health Care Financing Administration, "National Health Expenditures, 1986–2000," *Health Care Financing Review*, 8:4 (Summer 1987), p. 32.

Table 7. John Holahan and John L. Palmer, "Medicare's Fiscal Problems: An Imperative for Reform." Reprinted with permission from *Journal of Health Politics, Policy and Law*, 13:1. Copyright © 1988 by Duke University Press.

Figure 1. Division of National Cost Estimates, Office of the Actuary, Health Care Financing Administration, "National Health Expenditures, 1986–2000," *Health Care Financing Review*, 8:4 (Summer 1987), p. 11.

Figure 2. National Institutes of Health, *NIH Data Book: 1988* (Bethesda: National Institutes of Health, 1989).

Figure 3. George A. Kaplan et al., "Socioeconomic Status and Health," in Robert W. Amler and H. Bruce Dull, eds., *Closing the Gap: The Burden of Unnecessary Illness* (New York: Oxford University Press, 1987). Reprinted with permission of Oxford University Press.

# NOTES

1.  Robert J. Blendon, "Three Systems: A Comparative Study," *Health Management Quarterly [HMQ]*, XI (First Quarter 1989), p. 3. Remarkably also, a majority (61 percent) said that they would prefer the Canadian system to our own.

1.  Web Ruble, "Rockwood Boy, 7, Loses Battle with Leukemia," *The Oregonian* (December 3, 1987), pp. A1 and A24.

2.  John Kitzhaber, "Who'll Live, Who'll Die?" *The Sunday Oregonian* (November 29, 1987), p. B1.

3.  Louis Harris, *Inside America* (New York: Vintage Books, 1987), p. 40; see also Arthur J. Barsky, *Worried Sick: Our Troubled Quest for Wellness* (Boston: Little, Brown, 1988), p. 80, on the paradox of "doing better, feeling worse."

4.  While he does not directly deal with the issues I discuss in this book, I was greatly stimulated to think of the idea of a "way of life" by Stuart Hampshire, *Morality and Conflict* (Cambridge: Harvard University Press, 1984).

# CHAPTER 2

1.  The discussion which follows on the definition is based on an earlier article of mine, Daniel Callahan, "The WHO Definition of Health," *Hastings Center Studies*, I:3 (1973), pp. 77–87.

2.  Cf. David Gauthier, "Unequal Need: A Problem of Equity in Access to Health Care," in President's Commission for the Study of Ethical Problems in Medicine and Biomedical and Behavioral Research, *Securing Access to Health Care*, Vol. 2, "The Ethical Implications of Differences in the Availability of Health Services" (Washington, D.C.: Government Printing Office, 1983), p. 180; Norman Daniels, *Just Health*

*Care* (New York: Cambridge University Press, 1989), p. 29; Callahan, op. cit., *passim*.

3. See Leon R. Kass, *Toward a More Natural Science: Biology and Human Affairs* (New York: The Free Press, 1985), especially pp. 164–174; Arthur L. Caplan, H. Tristram Engelhardt, Jr., and James J. McCartney, eds., *Concepts of Health and Disease: Interdisciplinary Perspectives* (Reading, Mass.: Addison-Wesley Publishing Co., 1981); Lennart Nordenfeldt, *On the Nature of Health* (Dordrecht, Holland: D. Reidel Publishing Co., 1987).

4. H. Tristram Engelhardt, Jr., in *The Foundations of Bioethics* (New York: Oxford University Press, 1986), develops this idea at great length; it is also taken up, critically, by Alasdair MacIntyre in *After Virtue* (Notre Dame, Ind.: University of Notre Dame Press, 1981); a good discussion of the general issues can be found in Michael Senebel, ed., *Liberalism and Its Critics* (New York: New York University Press, 1984).

5. See especially Nordenfeldt, op. cit., pp. 57–70, for a good survey of various senses of "need"; David Wiggins and Siva Dermen, "Needs, Need, Needing," *Journal of Medical Ethics*, 13 (1987), pp. 62–68; David Braybrooke, *Meeting Needs* (Princeton: Princeton University Press, 1987).

6. I am adapting these definitions from a useful article by the Committee on Policy for DNR Decisions, Yale New Haven Hospital, "Report on Do Not Resuscitate Decisions," *Connecticut Medicine*, 47 (August 1983), p. 480.

7. Allen Buchanan, "The Right to a Decent Minimum of Health Care," in *Securing Access to Health Care*, Vol. 2, pp. 207–238; Anita F. Savvo, "Determining Medical Necessity Within Medicaid: A Proposal for Statutory Reform," *Nebraska Law Review*, 63 (1984), pp. 835–858; Howard H. Hiatt, *America's Health in the Balance: Choice or Chance?* (New York: Harper & Row, 1987), pp. 212–215; Norman Daniels, op. cit., pp. 26–28; Mary N. Baily, "Rationing Medical Care: Processes for Defining Adequacy," and David D. Friedman, "Comments on 'Rationing Medical Care: Processes for Defining Adequacy,' " in George J. Agich and Charles E. Begley, eds., *The Price of Health* (Dordrecht, Holland: D. Reidel Publishing Co., 1986), pp. 165–197.

8. President's Commission, *Securing Access to Health Care*, Vol. I, p. 22.

9. While the Commission seemed to cast doubt on the utility of the concept of "needs" its analysis appeared to presume its value; see Larry R. Churchill, *Rationing Health Care in America: Perceptions and Principles of Justice* (Notre Dame, Ind.: University of Notre Dame Press, 1987), p. 97. It is, in fact, hard to see how there can be any coherent notion of a minimal, or necessary, or adequate level of care without some concept of individual need to give it content.

10. There are a number of interesting and valuable discussions of the problems, theoretical and practical, in trying to define "needs" for policy purposes. See especially Ruth Macklin, "Equal Access to Professional Services: Medicine," *Journal of Professional and Business Ethics*,

4 (Spring/Summer 1985), pp. 1–12; "Commentary," by Bruce Jennings, *Journal of Professional and Business Ethics*, 4 (Spring/Summer 1985), pp. 13–24; Jeffrey Hadorn, "Creating a Just and Affordable System of National Health Insurance," unpublished M.A. thesis, 1988, University of Colorado; Gerald R. Winslow, *Triage and Justice* (Berkeley: University of California Press, 1982), pp. 41–42; Gene Outka, "Social Justice and Equal Access to Health Care," *Journal of Religious Ethics*, 2:1 (Spring 1974), pp. 11–32; Ronald Bayer et al., "Toward Justice in Health Care," *American Journal of Public Health*, 78: 5 (May 1988), esp. p. 586; Paul T. Menzel, *Medical Costs, Moral Choices: A Philosophy of Health Care Economics in America* (New Haven: Yale University Press, 1983), pp. 81–85; Earl E. Shelp, ed., *Justice and Health Care* (Dordrecht, Holland: D. Reidel Publishing Co., 1981), *passim*; David T. Ozar, "What Should Count as Basic Health Care?" *Theoretical Medicine*, 4: 2 (June 1983), pp. 129–141; Robert P. Rhodes, "Optimizing Health: Why Equality of Access to Health Care Based on Need Leads to Injustice,"in David H. Smith, ed., *Respect and Care in Medical Ethics* (Lanham, Md.: University Press of America, 1984), p. 187; Jerry Avorn, "Needs, Wants, Demands, and Interests: Their Interaction in Medical Practice and Health Policy," in Ronald Bayer et al., eds., *In Search of Equity: Health Needs and the Health Care System* (New York: Plenum Press, 1983), pp. 185ff.; Robert G. Evans, *Strained Mercy: The Economics of Canadian Health Care* (Toronto: Butterworth & Co., 1984), pp. 21–26.

11. Charles Fried, "Equality and Rights in Medical Care," *Hastings Center Report*, 6 (February 1976), p. 32.

12. Renée C. Fox, *The Courage to Fail: A Social View of Organ Transplants and Dialysis* (Chicago: University of Chicago Press, 2nd. ed., 1978), esp. Chap. 8, pp. 226–265.

13. For some general writings on cost-benefit and cost-effectiveness analysis, see M. C. Weinstein and W. B. Stason, "Foundation of Cost-Effectiveness Analysis for Health and Medical Practices," *New England Journal of Medicine*, 296 (1977), pp. 716–721; E. J. Mishan, *Cost-Benefit Analysis* (New York: Praeger, 1976); Jerry Avorn has shown how a use of cost-benefit analysis could work against the elderly in "Benefit and Cost Analysis in Geriatric Care," *New England Journal of Medicine*, 310 (May 17, 1984), pp. 1294–1301.

14. An excellent analysis of the strengths and weaknesses of QALYS can be found in Paul Menzel, *Strong Medicine* (New York: Oxford University Press, forthcoming 1989), Chap. 5; see also "Logic in Medicine: An Economic Perspective," *British Medical Journal*, 295 (December 12, 1987), pp. 1537–1541; Alan Williams, "Economics of Coronary Artery Bypass Grafting," *British Medical Journal*, 291 (August 3, 1985), pp. 326–329; Michael O'Donnell, "One Man's Burden," *British Medical Journal*, 293 (July 5, 1986), p. 59; a response by Alan Williams to O'Donnell, *British Medical Journal*, 293 (August 2, 1986), pp. 337–338; John Harris, "QALYfying the Value of Life," *Journal of Medical Ethics*, 13 (1987), pp. 117–123. For a valuable discussion of the problems of selecting patients for scarce treatment in the absence of clear criteria, see Janet F. Haas, "Admission to Rehabilitation Centers: Selection of Pa-

tients," *Archives of Physical Medicine and Rehabilitation*, 69 (May 1988), pp. 1–26. One reason the British National Health Service has managed to control costs is that physicians and other experts have defined need, not patients. But this was simply a shift of power, and a political act, a point nicely made in Rudolf Klein's fascinating study of the relationship between need and demand in England, *The Politics of the National Health Service* (London: Longman, 1983), pp. 158–160.

15.     Braybrooke, op. cit., p. 301.

16.     The idea of normal species functioning is elegantly developed in Daniels, *Just Health Care*, pp. 26ff.

17.     Office of Disease Prevention and Health Promotion, "Mental Illness," in *Disease Prevention/Health Promotion* (Palo Alto: Bull Publishing Co., 1988), pp. 308–319.

18.     Quoted in Rudolf Klein, *The Politics of the National Health Service*, pp. 66–67.

19.     See Gregory de Lissovoy, "Medicare and Heart Transplants: Will Lightning Strike Twice?" *Health Affairs*, 7 (Fall 1988), pp. 61–72; see also L. Henry Edmunds et al., "Open Heart Surgery in Octogenarians," *New England Journal of Medicine*, 319 (July 21, 1988), pp. 131–135.

20.     Arthur J. Barsky, *Worried Sick: Our Troubled Quest for Wellness* (Boston: Little, Brown, 1988), p. 187.

21.     Elizabeth Royte, "Being Rich," *Self* (November 1988), p. 154.

22.     See Paul Menzel, *Medical Costs, Medical Choices*, p. 82.

23.     For a good discussion of the idea of a "right to health care" see James F. Childress, "Rights to Health Care in a Democratic Society," in James M. Humber and Robert Almeder, eds., *Biomedical Ethics Review, 1984* (Clifton, N. J.: Humana Press, 1984), pp. 47–70; John D. Arras, "Utility, Natural Rights, and the Right to Health Care," *Biomedical Ethics Review, 1984*, pp. 47–70; "Rights to Health Care," a special issue of *The Journal of Medicine and Philosophy*, 4 (June 1979). Also of great interest is Robert M. Veatch, *The Foundations of Justice* (New York: Oxford University Press, 1986.)

24.     The United Nations Universal Declaration of Human Rights, Article 25. I.

25.     Statement of the American Medical Association to the Subcommittee on Health, Committee on Finance, United States Senate, July 29, 1988.

26.     Henry Shue, *Basic Rights: Subsistence, Affluence, and U.S. Foreign Policy* (Princeton: Princeton University Press, 1980), pp. 24–25.

27.     There have also been long-standing doubts about the validity of positive, welfare rights. See Alasdair MacIntyre, "The Right to Die Garrulously," in Richard L. Purtell, ed., *Moral Dilemmas: Readings in Ethics and Social Philosophy* (Belmont: Wadsworth Publishing Co., 1985), pp. 129–134.

28.     Two interesting articles analyze the shift of the President's Commission from the language of rights to that of obligation: Ronald Bayer, "Ethics, Politics, and Access to Health Care," *Cardozo Law Review*, 6 (1984), pp. 303–320; John Arras, "Retreat from the Right to Health Care," *Cardozo Law Review*, 6 (1984), pp. 321–345.

29.     Health Care Financing Administration, *Special Report: Findings from the National Kidney Dialysis and Kidney Transplantation Study* (Baltimore: U.S. Department of Health and Human Services, 1987); see also Alonzo L. Plough, *Borrowed Time: Artificial Organs and the Politics of Extending Lives* (Philadelphia: Temple University Press, 1986).

30.     Robert A. Gutman, "High-Cost Life Prolongation: The National Kidney Dialysis and Kidney Transplantation Study," *Annals of Internal Medicine*, 108 (June 1988), p. 899.

31.     de Lissovoy, op. cit., p. 72.

32.     Bruce Jennings, Daniel Callahan, and Arthur L. Caplan, "Ethical Challenges of Chronic Illness," *Hastings Center Report*, Special Supplement (February/March 1988), pp. 1–16; Anselm L. Strauss et al., *Chronic Illness and the Quality of Life* (St. Louis: C.V. Mosby Co., 2nd ed., 1984).

CHAPTER 3

1.      Informative discussions of the general problems of the U.S. healthcare "system" can be found in Eli Ginzberg, "The Destabilization of Health Care," *New England Journal of Medicine*, 315 (September 18, 1986), pp. 757–760; Robert L. Dickman et al., "An End to Patchwork Reform of Health Care," *New England Journal of Medicine*, 317 (October 22, 1987), pp. 1086–1089.

2.      See *National Health Insurance: Major Proposals*, Hearings before the United States House of Representatives, December 8–10, 1975 (Washington, D.C.: Government Printing Office, Serial No. 94–60, 1976); Paul Starr, *The Social Transformation of American Medicine* (New York: Basic Books, 1982), *passim*.

3.      A characteristic description of this kind can be found in the excellent study by Robert J. Rubin et al., *Critical Condition: America's Health Care in Jeopardy* (Washington, D.C.: National Committee for Quality Health Care, 1988), p. 1.

4.      Uwe E. Reinhardt, "U.S. Health Policy: Errors of Youth," *The Generational Journal* (April 1988), p. 44.

5.      Office of Technology Assessment, *Healthy Children: Investing in the Future* (Washington, D.C.: Office of Technology Assessment, 1988), pp. 41–44; see also The Robert Wood Johnson Foundation, *Access to Health Care in the United States: Results of a 1986 Survey* (Princeton, N.J.: The Robert Wood Johnson Foundation, 1986); see also Timothy H. Smeeding and Barbara Boyld Torrey, "Poor Children in Rich Countries," *Science*, 242 (November 11, 1988), pp. 873–877.

6. Charles N. Oberg and Cynthia Longseth Polich, "Medicaid: Entering the Third Decade," *Health Affairs* (Fall 1988), p. 91.

7. "Long Term Care and Personal Impoverishment: Seven in Ten Elderly Living Alone Are at Risk," *A Report Presented by the Chairman of the Select Committee on Aging, U.S. House of Representatives* (Washington, D.C.: Government Printing Office, Comm. Pub. No. 100–631, 1987).

8. Alice M. Rivlin and Joshua M. Wiener, *Caring for the Disabled Elderly: Who Will Pay?* (Washington, D.C.: The Brookings Institution, 1988), pp. 210ff.

9. Cf. Uwe E. Reinhardt, "Somber Clouds on the Horizon," *Health Week Forecast '88* (December 23, 1987), p. 6.

10. Gerald F. Anderson and Jane E. Erickson, "National Medical Care Spending," *Health Affairs* (Fall 1987), pp. 96–112.

11. Glenn Kramon, "A Few Expensive Procedures Are Focus of Effort to Trim Bill," *New York Times* (February 18, 1988), p. D1.

12. An excellent summary of developments over the past few decades can be found in Lawrence D. Brown, "Introduction to a Decade in Transition," *Journal of Health Politics, Policy and Law*, 11 (1986), pp. 569–583.

13. Joseph Califano has many interesting things to say about corporate cost-containment efforts in *America's Health Care Revolution* (New York: Random House, 1986).

14. See Stephen H. Long and W. Pete Welch, "Are We Containing Costs or Pushing on a Balloon? *Health Affairs* (Fall 1988), pp. 113–117. They show, as do other studies, that we have done worse during the 1980s— at a time of greatly increased cost-containment efforts—than during the 1970s; see also Gerard F. Anderson and Jane E. Erickson, "National Medical Care Spending," *Health Affairs* (Fall 1987), pp. 96–112.

15. A sober assessment is provided by Harvey M. Sapolsksy, "Prospective Payment in Perspective," *Journal of Health Politics, Policy and Law*, 11 (1986), pp. 633–645.

16. See, for instance, James C. Robinson et al., "Hospital Competition and Surgical Length of Stay," *Journal of the American Medical Association*, 259 (February 5, 1988), pp. 696–700; James C. Robinson, "Competition and the Cost of Hospital Care, 1972–1982," *Journal of the American Medical Association*, 257 (June 19, 1987), pp. 3241–3245; D. Farley, *Competition Among Hospitals: Market Structure and Its Relation to Utilization, Costs, and Financial Position*, Research Note 7, U.S. Department of Health and Human Services, National Center for Health Services Research, Hospital Cost and Utilization Project (Washington, D.C.: Department of Health and Human Services, 1985); Stuart H. Altman, "Can We Control Health-Care Costs?" *Health Management Quarterly*, 10 (First Quarter 1988), pp. 15–19; Carl J. Schramm, "Revisiting the Competition/ Regulation Debate in Health Care Cost Containment," *Inquiry*, 23 (Fall 1986), pp. 236–242; George J. Agich and Charles E. Begley, "Some Problems with Pro-Competition Reforms," *Social Science and Medicine*, 21 (1985), pp. 623–630; Warren Greenberg, ed., "Special Issue on

Competition in the Health Care Sector: Ten Years Later," *Journal of Health Politics, Policy and Law*, 13: 2 (Summer 1988). In an afterword, commenting on the papers in the special issue, Lawrence D. Brown concludes that "all the authors have agreed that since 1978 we have made substantial progress toward enhancing competition . . . but remarkably, none shows—or even contends—that this progress has saved the system money" (p. 362); a more hopeful note is struck in Robert C. Bradbury, "A Community Approach to Health Care Competition," *Inquiry*, 24 (Fall 1987), pp. 253–265.

17.   See Jeffrey Merrill and Catherine McLaughlin, "Competition versus Regulation: Some Empirical Evidence," *Journal of Health Politics, Policy and Law*, 10 (Winter 1986), pp. 613–623; Catherine G. McLaughlin, Jeffrey C. Merrill, and Andrew J. Freed, "The Impact of HMO Growth on Hospital Costs and Utilization," in Richard Scheffler and Louis Rossiter, eds., *Advances in Health Economics and Health Services Research*, Vol. 5 (Greenwich, Conn.: JAI Press, 1984); Harold S. Luft, "How Do Health Maintenance Organizations Achieve Their 'Savings'?" *New England Journal of Medicine*, 298 (June 15, 1978), pp. 1336–1343; Willard Manning et al., "A Controlled Trial of a Prepaid Group Practice on Use of Services," *New England Journal of Medicine*, 310 (June 7, 1984), pp. 1505–1510; Eli Ginzberg, "A Hard Look at Cost Containment," *New England Journal of Medicine*, 316 (April 30, 1987), p. 1152; Milton Freudenheim, "Prepaid Programs for Health Care Encounter Snags," *New York Times* (January 31, 1988), p. 1.

18.   The first state to adopt the DRG system was New Jersey, in 1980. William C. Hsaio and Daniel L. Dunn, "The Impact of DRG Payment on New Jersey Hospitals," *Inquiry*, 24 (Fall 1987), pp. 212–220; Ginzberg, "A Hard Look at Cost Containment," Paul C. Rettig et al., "Medicare's Prospective Payment: Some Retrospective Observations," *New England Journal of Medicine*, 318 (June 23, 1988), pp. 1681–1683; Judith Feder, Jack Hadley, and Stephen Zuckerman, *A Statistical Analysis of the Effects of Medicare's Prospective Payment System on Hospitals* (Washington, D.C.: The Urban Institute, June 1987); Stephen H. Long and W. Pete Welch, op. cit., p. 117. A much more optimistic study concludes that the DRG prospective payment plan has had a significant impact: Louise B. Russell and Carrie Lynn Manning, "The Effect of Prospective Payment on Medicare Expenditure," *New England Journal of Medicine*, 320 (February 16, 1989), pp. 439–444; see also *Medicare Prospective Payment and the American Health Care System* (Washington, D.C.: Prospective Payment Commission, 1988), which also concludes that it has slowed the growth of medical expenditures.

19.   Alain C. Enthoven, "Managed Competition: An Agenda for Action," *Health Affairs*, 7 (Summer 1988), p. 28. The entire issue of the journal is given over to "The Managed Care Revolution."

20.   For a relatively optimistic view, see Paul J. Feldstein, Thomas C. Wickizer, and John A. C. Wheeler, "Private Cost Containment: The Effects of Utilization Review Programs on Health Care Use and Expenditures," *New England Journal of Medicine*, 318 (May 19, 1988), pp. 1310–1313; but see also Samuel A. Mitchell and John R. Virts, "Health Care Cost

Containment: What Is Enough?" *Health Affairs,* 5 (Winter 1986), who argue that it is dangerous to assume there is "too much fluff" in the U.S. system (pp. 112–113).

21. Ginzberg, "A Hard Look . . . ," p. 1154; William B. Schwartz, "The Inevitable Failure of Current Cost-Containment Strategies," *Journal of the American Medical Association,* 257 (January 9, 1987), pp. 220–224.

22. See especially Dorothy P. Rice and Mitchell LaPlante, "Chronic Illness, Disability, and Increasing Longevity," in Sean Sullivan and Marion Ein Lewis, eds., *The Economics and Ethics of Long-Term Care and Disability* (Washington, D.C.: American Enterprise Institute, 1988), pp. 9–55; also Lois M. Verbugge, "Longer Life but Worsening Health? Trends in Health and Mortality of Middle-Aged and Older Persons," *Milbank Memorial Fund Quarterly* (Fall 1984), pp. 475–519; Kenneth G. Manton, "Changing Concepts of Morbidity and Mortality in the Elderly Population," *Milbank Memorial Fund Quarterly* (Spring 1982), pp. 183–244.

23. Grant E. Steffen, "Quality Medical Care: A Definition," *Journal of the American Medical Association,* 260 (July 1, 1988), pp. 56–61.

24. See Health Care Quality Alliance, *Quality Health Care: Critical Issues Before the Nation* (no place of publication given, March 1988); Lewin and Associates, "Quality of Care: Summary of Major Research Projects in Progress" (no place of publication given, November 1987).

25. Philip Caper, "Defining Quality in Medical Care," *Health Affairs,* 7 (Spring 1988), esp. pp. 52–53; in addition, the entire issue of *Health Affairs* in which the Caper article appears is devoted to the topic of "The Pursuit of Quality"; also, a special issue of another journal: "The Challenge of Quality" in *Inquiry,* 25 (Spring 1988); Uwe E. Reinhardt, "Quality Assessment of Medical Care: An Economist's Perspective," *QRB* (September 1983), pp. 252–257.

26. Wendy L. Wall, "Cost Cuts Are Seen Hurting Health Care," *Wall Street Journal* (April 28, 1988), p. 26; Stephen H. Shortell and Edward F. X. Hughes, "The Effects of Regulation, Competition, and Ownership on Mortality Rates Among Hospital Inpatients," *New England Journal of Medicine,* 318 (April 28, 1988), pp. 1100–1107; *AMN* staff, "DRGs, PROs Adversely Affecting Patient Care," *American Medical News* (March 18, 1988), p. 34; in a more theoretical vein, Victor Fuchs, "Has Cost Containment Gone Too Far?" *Milbank Memorial Quarterly,* 64 (1986), p. 331ff; Victor Cohn, "Going Home Too Soon—Or Too Sick," *Washington Post* (July 5, 1988), p. 10; Robert J. Blendon and David E. Rogers, "Cutting Medical Care Costs: *Primum Non Nocere,*" *Journal of the American Medical Association,* 250 (October 14, 1983), pp. 1880–1885.

27. A helpful discussion of the role of American values and institutions in exacerbating cost-containment and rationing problems can be found in Robert H. Blank, *Rationing Medicine* (New York: Columbia University Press, 1988), esp. Chap. 4, "The Role of Government Institutions"; see also Maxwell J. Mehlman, "Rationing Expensive Life Saving Medical Treatments," *Wisconsin Law Review,* 2 (1985), pp. 239–303, for a discussion of all the legal objections that could be directed at rationing schemes.

28.    Robert J. Rubin et al., op. cit., p. vii.

29.    See Uwe E. Reinhardt, "Resource Allocation in Health Care: The Allocation of Lifestyles to Providers," *Milbank Quarterly*, 65 (1987), pp. 153–176; David V. Himmelstein and Steffie Woolhandler, "Cost Without Benefit: Administrative Waste in U.S. Health Care," *New England Journal of Medicine*, 314 (February 13, 1986), pp. 441–445.

30.    Louis Harris and Associates, *Making Difficult Health Care Decisions* (Cambridge: The Loran Commission, June 1987), p. 5.

31.    Ibid.

32.    Ibid.

33.    Ibid., p. 115.

34.    Keith Melville and John Doble, *The Public's Perspective on Social Welfare Reform* (New York: The Public Agenda Foundation, January 1988).

35.    Ibid., p. 67.

36.    Ibid., p. 73; comparable results are reported in Gene Pokorny, "Report Card on Care in Health Care," *HMQ: Health Management Quarterly*, X (First Quarter 1988), p. 5.

37.    Robert G. Blendon and Drew E. Altman, "Public Attitudes about Health-Care Costs," *New England Journal of Medicine*, 311 (August 30, 1984), p. 614; but see also a new study by Blendon, "Three Systems: A Comparative Survey," *Health Management Quarterly*, XI (First Quarter 1989), pp. 2–10.

38.    Robert G. Evans, "Illusions of Necessity: Evading Responsibility for Choice in Health Care," *Journal of Health Politics, Policy and Law*, 10 (Fall 1985), pp. 439–467.

39.    An interesting discussion of the problem of attempting to carry the Canadian system and values to the United States can be found in Victor Fuchs, "Learning from the Canadian Experience," *Health Affairs*, 7 (Winter 1988), pp. 25–30; see also Robert G. Evans, "Split Vision: Interpreting Cross-Border Differences in Health Spending," *Health Affairs*, 7 (Winter 1988), pp. 17–24; Robert G. Evans et al., "Controlling Health Expenditures—The Canadian Reality," *New England Journal of Medicine*, 320 (March 2, 1989), pp. 571–577.

40.    Jean de Kervasdoue, John R. Kimberly, and Victor G. Rodwin, eds., *The End of an Illusion* (Berkeley: University of California Press, 1984), p. xviii.

41.    George J. Schieber and Jean-Pierre Poulier, "International Health Spending and Utilization Trends," *Health Affairs*, 7 (Fall 1988).

42.    Robert G. Evans, " 'We'll Take Care of It for You'—Health Care in the Canadian Community," *Daedalus*, 117 (Fall 1988), p. 185.

43.    Louis P. Garrison, Jr., and Gail R. Wilensky, "Cost Containment and Incentives for Technology," *Health Affairs*, 5 (Summer 1986), pp. 46–58.

44.    Robert G. Evans, "Illusions of Necessity . . . ," p. 453.

45.  The National Committee for Quality Health Care, *Medical Technology in the Competitive Market* (no place of publication given, February 1987), p. 4.

46.  Ibid., p. 2.4.

47.  Ibid., p. 2.5.

48.  Office of Technology Assessment, *Strategies of Medical Technology Assessment* (Washington D.C.: Government Printing Office, 1982), p. 3.

49.  A thorough discussion of medical technology assessment can be found in Institute of Medicine, *Assessing Medical Technologies* (Washington, D.C.: National Academy Press, 1985); see also Susan Bartlett Foote, "Assessing Medical Technology Assessment: Past, Present, and Future," *The Milbank Quarterly*, 65 (1987), pp. 59–80; Seymour Perry, "Technology Assessment: Continuing Uncertainty," *New England Journal of Medicine*, 314 (January 23, 1986), pp. 240–243.

50.  For an unusually interesting and perceptive study of the array of forces working against an effective use of technology assessment, see Barbara Koenig, "The Technological Imperative in Medical Practice: The Social Creation of (Routine) Treatment," in Margaret Lock and Deborah Gordon, eds., *Biomedicine Examined* (Dordrecht: Kluwer Academic Publishers, 1988), pp. 465–496; Ian Kennedy, *Treat Me Right: Essays in Medical Law and Ethics* (Oxford: Oxford University Press, 1988), pp. 287–299.

51.  Albert R. Jonsen, "Bentham in a Box: Technology Assessment and Health Care Allocation," *Law, Medicine and Health Care*, 14 (1986), pp. 172–174.

52.  Bryan Jennett, "Assessment of Clinical Technologies," *International Journal of Technology Assessment in Health Care*, 4 (1988), p. 437; see also Bryan Jennett, *High Technology Medicine: Benefits and Burdens* (London: Nuffield Provincial Hospitals Trust, 1982); Bryan Jennett, "High Technology Medicine: How Defined and How Regarded," *Milbank Memorial Fund Quarterly*, 63 (1985), pp. 141–173; M. Janet Barger-Lux and Robert P. Heaney, "For Better and Worse: The Technological Imperative in Health Care," *Social Science and Medicine*, 22 (1986), pp. 1313–1320.

53.  Gregory de Lissovoy, "Medicare and Heart Transplants: Will Lightning Strike Twice?" *Health Affairs* (Fall 1988), p. 70; see also de Lissovoy, "Patient Selection in the Medicare End-Stage Renal Disease Program," *Medical Care*, 26 (October 1988), pp. 959–970.

54.  See Stuart H. Altman, "Impact of the Changing Medical Payment System on Technological Innovation and Utilization," from Institute of Medicine, *New Medical Devices: Invention, Development, and Use* (Washington, D.C.: National Academy Press, 1988), who worries about cost-containment incentives so strong that they hinder the use of effective technologies.

55.  Maurice McGregor, "Technology and the Allocation of Resources," *New England Journal of Medicine*, 320 (January 12, 1989), p. 119. Dr. McGregor is one of the few analysts to have noted that it is success, not failure, that drives up costs; see also Robert J. Maxwell, *Health and*

*Wealth: An International Study of Health Care Spending* (Lexington, Mass.: D. C. Heath & Co., 1981), esp. his judgment that "the more successful medicine is with one set of problems, the more intractable the next set is likely to be" (p. 46).

56. Schwartz, op. cit., p. 223; see also the earlier, groundbreaking study, Henry J. Aaron and William B. Schwartz, *The Painful Prescription: Rationing Health Care* (Washington, D.C.: The Brookings Institution, 1984).

57. Alliance for Aging Research, *Aging Research on the Threshold of Discovery* (Washington, D.C.: Alliance for Aging Research, October 1987), p. 3.

58. See Rice and La Plante, op. cit.; Dorothy M. Gilford, ed., *The Aging Population in the Twenty-first Century* (Washington, D.C.: National Academy Press, 1988), esp. Chap. 4.

59. National Institutes of Health, *NIH Data Book: 1988* (Bethesda, Md.: National Institutes of Health, 1988), p. 1.

60. Ibid.; see also Chase N. Peterson, "The Costs of Biomedical Research," p. 87, Henry J. Aaron, "Questioning the Cost of Biomedical Research," pp. 96ff. in *Health Affairs* (Summer 1986).

61. For a powerful formulation of this point, drawing especially on the Canadian experiences, see Evans, "Lessons from Cost Containment," p. 597.

62. A balanced and helpful discussion can be found in Lawrence D. Brown, *Health Policy in the United States: Issues and Options* (New York: The Ford Foundation, 1988), pp. 8ff.

63. Steven A. Garfinkel, Gerald F. Riley, and Vincent G. Iannacchione, "High-Cost Users of Medical Care," *Health Care Financing Review*, 9 (Summer 1988), pp. 41–52.

64. Willard Gaylin, personal communication.

CHAPTER 4

1. For an interesting discussion of cultural differences in responding to illness, see Lynn Payer, *Medicine and Culture* (New York: Henry Holt, 1988); also Susan Barr, *Hypochondria: Woeful Imaginings* (Berkeley: University of California Press, 1988), esp. Chaps. 8 and 9 on hypochondria and cultural differences.

2. Cf. James F. Blumstein, "Thinking about Government's Role in Medical Care," *St. Louis University Law Journal*, 32 (1988), p. 860.

3. The best account of the deleterious effects of an excessive focus on health is to be found in Arthur J. Barsky, *Worried Sick: Our Troubled Quest for Wellness* (Boston, Little, Brown, 1988); see also Alvan R. Feinstein, "Scientific Standards in Epidemiologic Studies of the Menace of Daily Life," *Science*, 242 (December 4, 1988), pp. 1257–1263, for a discussion of data on supposed health menaces.

4. Dorothy P. Rice and Mitchell P. LaPlante, "Chronic Illness, Disability, and Increasing Longevity," in Sean Sullivan and Marion Ein Lewin, eds., *The Economics and Ethics of Long-Term Care and Disability* (Washington, D.C.: American Enterprise Institute, 1988), p. 20. A useful discussion of earlier patterns of national spending on health in relationship to other needs can be found in "Special Study on Economic Change," Vol. 6 of *Federal Finance: The Pursuit of American Goals* (Washington, D.C.: Joint Economic Committee, Congress of the United States, 1980).

5. This problem is discussed in an informative way in Peter G. Peterson and Neil Howe, *On Borrowed Time* (San Francisco: Institute for Contemporary Studies, 1988), esp. p. 59 and p. 169. Rudolph Klein makes the telling point that, in England, "by rejecting an insurance-based health service . . . the founders of the NHS [National Health Service] ensured that it would have to compete with other government departments for general tax-revenue: with education, housing and all other claims for resources," *The Politics of the National Health Service* (London: Longman, 1983), p. 37.

6. See, for example, National Research Council, *Everybody Counts: A Report to the Nation on the Future of Mathematics Education* (Washington, D.C.: National Academy Press, 1989).

7. Dorothy P. Rice et al., "The Economic Costs of Illness: A Replication and Update," *Health Care Financing Review*, 7 (Fall 1985), pp. 61–80; Thomas A. Hodgson, "The State of the Art of Cost-of-Illness Estimates," *Advances in Health Economics and Health Services Research*, 4 (1983), pp. 129–164.

8. Barsky, op. cit., pp. 83–87.

9. Paul Ramsey, *The Patient as Person* (New Haven: Yale University Press, 1970), p. 240.

10. Uwe Reinhardt, "The Macroeconomic Vision of Cost Containment," *Hospitals* (February 20, 1988), p. 20.

11. Uwe Reinhardt, "The Best Defense: Argue Outputs, Not Jobs," *Hospitals* (April 20, 1988), p. 17.

12. Uwe Reinhardt, "What Percentage of the GNP Should Be Spent on Health?", unpublished paper, January 1983, p. 9. I am indebted to Lester Thurow, Ruth Hanft, Victor R. Fuchs, and Uwe Reinhardt for some helpful correspondence on these issues.

13. Lester Carl Thurow, "Learning to Say 'No,' " *New England Journal of Medicine*, 311 (December 13, 1984), p. 1569.

14. Stuart H. Altman, "Impact of the Changing Medical Payment System on Technological Innovation and Utilization," in National Academy of Sciences, *New Medical Devices: Invention, Development, and Use* (Washington, D.C.: National Academy of Sciences, 1988), p. 93.

15. Herbert Stein, "The Real Deficits—and Surpluses," *The Economist* (June 1988), p. 2; Stein, *Governing the 5 Trillion Dollar Economy* (New York: Oxford University Press, 1989).

16. Ibid., p. 7.

17. Thurow, op. cit., p. 1572.

18. Victor R. Fuchs, *Who Shall Live? Health, Economics and Social Choice* (New York: Basic Books, 1974), p. 20; see also Victor R. Fuchs, "Has Cost Containment Gone Too Far?" *The Milbank Quarterly*, 64 (1986), pp. 479–488.

19. Organization for Economic Cooperation and Development, *Financing and Delivering Health Care*, OECD Social Policy Studies No. 4 (Paris: OECD, 1987), p. 45; Barsky, op. cit., p. 195.

20. Phillip Longman, *Born to Pay: The New Politics of Aging in America* (Boston: Houghton Mifflin, 1987), p. 90.

21. I tried to consider this issue at length in another piece; see Daniel Callahan, "The Social Responsibility of Science in the Face of Uncertain Consequences," in *Ethical and Scientific Issues Posed by Human Uses of Molecular Genetics*, Annals of the New York Academy of Sciences, 265 (January 23, 1976), pp. 1–12.

CHAPTER 5

1. Two books of enduring value on the history of human health and medical developments are Thomas McKeown, *The Role of Medicine: Dream, Mirage, or Nemesis?* (Princeton, Princeton University Press, 1979); René Dubos, *Mirage of Health: Utopias, Progress and Biological Change* (New York: Harper Colophon Books, 1979).

2. Morton Kramer, "The Rising Pandemic of Mental Disorders and Associated Chronic Diseases and Disorders," *Acta Psychiatrica Scandinavica*, Suppl. 185, Vol. 62 (1980), pp. 382–396; Ernest M. Gruenberg, "The Failures of Success," *Milbank Memorial Fund Quarterly* (Winter 1977), pp. 3–24; Dorothy P. Rice and Mitchell P. LaPlante, "Chronic Illness, Disability, and Increasing Longevity," in Sean Sullivan and Marion Ein Lewin, eds., *The Economics and Ethics of Long-Term Care and Disability* (Washington, D.C.: American Enterprise Institute, 1988), pp. 9–55; Kenneth E. Manton, "Future Patterns of Chronic Disease Incidence, Disability, and Mortality Among the Elderly: Implications for the Demand for Acute and Long-Term Health Care," *New York State Journal of Medicine* (November 1985), pp. 623–633.

3. See James F. Fries, "Age, Illness, and Health Policy: Implications of the Compression of Morbidity," *Perspectives in Biology and Medicine*, 31 (Spring 1988), pp. 407–428, and Fries, "Reduction of the National Morbidity," *Gerontologica Perspecta*, 1 (1987), pp. 54–65.

4. See Lester C. Thurow, "Medicine versus Economics," *New England Journal of Medicine*, 313 (September 5, 1985), p. 614, on the need to change general attitudes in this respect.

5. Larry R. Churchill, *Rationing Health Care in America: Perceptions and Principles of Justice* (Notre Dame, Ind.: University of Notre Dame, 1987),

p. 103. I greatly profited from a reading of Leon R. Kass's paper "The Mentally Retarded Citizen and the Good Community," unpublished paper; for an effort to grapple with the problem of healthcare and utilitarianism, see Gavin Mooney and Alastair McGuire, *Medical Ethics and Economics in Health Care* (Oxford: Oxford University Press, 1988).

6.    One of the best discussions of suffering in a health context is Eric J. Cassell, "The Nature of Suffering and the Goals of Medicine," *New England Journal of Medicine*, 306 (March 18, 1982), pp. 639–645; see also Arthur Kleinman, *The Illness Narratives: Suffering, Healing and the Human Condition* (New York: Basic Books, 1988); Robert S. Downie and Elizabeth Telfer, *Caring and Curing* (New York: Methuen, 1980); Seymour B. Sarason, *Caring and Compassion in Clinical Practice* (San Francisco: Jossey-Bass, 1985).

7.    Leon Eisenberg, "The Search for Care," *Daedalus*, 106 (Winter 1977), pp. 237–238; Milton Mayeroff, *On Caring* (New York: Harper and Row, 1971); Willard Gaylin, *Caring* (New York: Alfred Knopf, 1976); Stanley Hauerwas, "Care," in Warren Reich, ed., *Encyclopedia of Bioethics* (New York: The Free Press, 1978), Vol. 1, pp. 145–150; Howard Brody, *Stories of Sickness* (New Haven: Yale University Press, 1987).

8.    Rudolf Klein, in *The Politics of the National Health Service* (London: Longman, 1983), has written, "Even if the limitations of medical technology in curing disease and disability are now becoming apparent, there are no such limitations on the scope of health services for providing care for those who cannot be cured" (p. 182). I think Klein seriously overstates the possibilities here. While demand for care can be quite elastic, it would not be *inherently* open-ended the way cure is. People can be comforted, even institutionally cared for, within an individual limit of expenditure not possible in advanced forms of constantly improved high-technology medicine. We can impose strong limits on individual caring and yet still provide decent care. We can give everyone a decent level of caring while we cannot, say, guarantee that we will be able to afford to save 200-gram babies and provide every 100-year-old with an artificial heart. The "intensity of service" that has been the principal source of inflationary healthcare costs beyond those brought by general inflation need not have an equivalent in caring. We could of course ruin this possibility by bringing high technology to caring in an intense fashion (e.g., total parenteral nutrition). Thus a reasonable set of limits on caring would include a limit on technological aids to caring, a requirement for substantial family caring, and resistance of an excessively high standard of "quality." A growing, and most likely, chronic shortage of people to provide caring, and the changing pattern of family life are, indeed, likely to themselves impose some limits—just as they will pose obstacles to providing decent care.

9.    See Bruce Jennings, Daniel Callahan, and Arthur L. Caplan, "Ethical Challenges of Chronic Illness," *Hastings Center Report*, Special Supplement (February/March 1988); Arthur Kleinman, op. cit.; Anselm L. Strauss et al., *Chronic Illness and the Quality of Life* (St. Louis: C.V. Mosby, 1984); Myron G. Eisenberg et al., eds., *Chronic Illness and Disability through the Life-Span* (New York: Springer Publishing Co., 1984);

Anselm Strauss and Juliet M. Corbin, *Shaping a New Health Care System* (San Francisco: Jossey-Bass, 1988).

10. Ray Fitzpatrick et al., *The Experience of Illness* (New York: Tavistock, 1984).

11. See especially James F. Fries, "The Future of the Health Care Professions: Implications of Changing Patterns of Mortality and Morbidity" (Stanford: Department of Medicine, Stanford University School of Medicine, 1988).

12. These matters have been most eloquently addressed by Leon R. Kass, *Toward a More Natural Science: Biology and Human Affairs* (New York: Free Press, 1985), and by Otto E. Guttentag, "The Meaning of Death in Medical Theory," *Stanford Medical Bulletin*, 17 (August 1959), pp. 165–170.

13. I have developed these ideas on healthcare and the elderly at length in Daniel Callahan, *Setting Limits: Medical Goals in an Aging Society* (New York: Simon and Schuster, 1987).

CHAPTER 6

1. Gerald F. Anderson and Jane E. Erickson, "National Medical Care Spending," *Health Affairs* (Fall 1987), p. 98.

2. The Working Group on Mechanical Circulatory Support of the National Heart, Lung, and Blood Institute, *Artificial Heart and Assist Devices: Directions, Needs, Costs, Societal and Ethical Issues* (Washington, D.C.: National Heart, Lung, and Blood Institute, May 1985). For data on dialysis, see Health Care Financing Administration, *Health Care Financing, Special Report: Findings from the National Kidney Dialysis and Kidney Transplantation Study* (Baltimore, Md.: U.S. Department of Health and Human Services, October 1987).

3. Barbara J. Culliton, "Politics of the Heart," *Science*, 241 (July 15, 1988), p. 283.

4. Maxwell J. Mehlman, "Health Care Cost Containment and Medical Technology: A Critique of Waste Theory," *Case Western Reserve Law Review*, 36 (1985–1986), p. 834.

5. For an analysis of this kind, looking at children who had earlier been treated in a neonatal intensive care unit, see Seetha Shankavan et al., "Medical Care Costs of High-Risk Infants After Neonatal Intensive Care: A Controlled Study," *Pediatrics*, 81 (March 1988), pp. 372–378.

6. For a particularly frank discussion of lobbying tactics to gain increased research funds, see David R. Hathaway, "Revitalizing the Federal Commitment in Support of Biomedical Research," *Clinical Research*, 36 (September 1988), pp. 475–482.

7. See Edward L. Schneider, "Options to Control the Rising Health Care Costs of Older Americans," *Journal of the American Medical Association*, 261 (February 10, 1989), pp. 907–908. It is a source of some mystery in

this respect why, as mortality declines, research investments continue to climb. Cardiovascular disease, for instance, has seen a 25 percent mortality decline since 1976, while the NIH research outlay of the National Heart, Lung and Blood Institute has more than doubled over the same period—see National Institutes of Health, *NIH Data Book: 1987* (Bethesda, Md.: National Institutes of Health, 1987).

8.  James F. Fries, "Aging, Illness, and Health Policy: Implications of the Compression of Morbidity," *Perspectives in Biology and Medicine*, 31 (Spring 1988), p. 408.

9.  See Edward L. Schneider and J. A. Brody, "Aging, Natural Death, and the Compression of Morbidity: Another View," *New England Journal of Medicine*, 309 (1983), pp. 854–856.

10. Fries, op. cit., p. 420.

11. Alexander Leaf, personal communication; the late Selma J. Mushkin showed how, in the mid-1970s, the NIH budget correlated heavily with the number of deaths from a disease, even though other health needs posed severe problems also: *Biomedical Research: Costs and Benefits* (Cambridge: Ballinger Publishing Co., 1979), esp. Chap. 6, "Biomedical Research Priorities and Death."

12. Although his book is very different from this one in its themes and emphases, I was greatly stimulated to think about a public health perspective by Dan E. Beauchamp, *The Health of the Republic* (Philadelphia: Temple University Press, 1988); see also Institute of Medicine, *The Future of Public Health* (Washington, D.C.: National Academy Press, 1988).

13. Ian Kennedy is correct, I believe, in saying that "medical treatment ought to be divided into two classes. The first we can call regular, standard, or ordinary treatment . . . the second we can call unusual, or special treatment, requiring more than ordinary skill, effort or resources . . . [such a division] is . . . essential for solving resource problems," in *Treat Me Right: Essays in Medical Law and Ethics* (Oxford: Clarendon Press, 1988), p. 292.

CHAPTER 7

1.  Rudolf Klein has an interesting discussion of this distinction in *The Politics of the National Health Service* (London: Longman, 1983), pp. 175–176.

2.  Robert G. Evans, "Finding the Levers, Finding the Courage: Lessons from Cost Containment in North America," *Journal of Health Politics, Policy and Law*, 11 (1986), p. 597.

3.  A particularly valuable study of an integrated system, that of British services for the elderly, can be found in William Halsey Barker, *Adding Life to Years: Organized Geriatrics Services in Great Britain and Implications for the United States* (Baltimore: Johns Hopkins University Press, 1987).

4. See Diana B. Dutton, *Worse than the Disease: Pitfalls of Medical Progress* (New York: Cambridge University Press, 1988), p. 368, for a summary of planning possibilities. See also Institute of Medicine, *DHEW's Research Planning Principles: A Review* (Washington, D.C.: National Academy of Sciences, 1979); Dorothy Nelkin, "Science and Technology Policy and the Democratic Process," *Studies in Science Education*, 9 (1982), pp. 47–64.

5. Lester Thurow has sketched a three-tier system in "Medicine versus Economics," *New England Journal of Medicine*, 313 (September 5, 1985), pp. 611–614.

6. For a strong defense of a one-tier system, see Amy Gutmann, "For and Against Equal Access to Health Care," President's Commission for the Study of Ethical Problems in Medicine and Biomedical and Behavioral Research, *Securing Access to Health Care*, Vol. 2 (Washington, D.C.: Government Printing Office, 1983), pp. 51–66.

7. See Louis Harris and Associates, *Making Difficult Health Care Decisions* (Cambridge: The Loran Commission, June 1987); John Melville and John Doble, *The Public's Perspective on Social Welfare Reform* (New York: The Public Agenda Foundation, 1988).

8. For an interesting discussion of changing attitudes toward taxation, see Peter T. Kilborn, "Tax System: Efficiency versus Fairness," *New York Times* (December 10, 1988), p. C1.

9. Business will, in any case, have its hands full with the proposed new accounting rules calling for a disclosure of liability for unfunded medical and insurance benefits of its retired workers, the so-called FASB Rule of the Financial Accounting Standards Board. Uwe Reinhardt has been persistent in pointing out that proposals to saddle business with the cost of a universal coverage plan are simply a form of disguised taxation: See, for instance, "Toward a Fail-Safe Health-Insurance Scheme," *Wall Street Journal* (January 11, 1989), p. A16, and "How to Finance Our Changing Health Care System," *Bulletin of the New York Academy of Medicine*, 63 (January/February 1987), pp. 7–19.

10. J. Wennberg and A. Gittleson, "Small Area Variations in Health Care Delivery," *Science*, 182 (1973), pp. 1102–1108; John Wennberg, "Which Rate Is Right?" *New England Journal of Medicine*, 314 (January 30, 1986), pp. 310–311.

11. Lee Goldman et al., "A Computer Protocol to Predict Myocardial Infarction in Emergency Department Patients with Chest Pain," *New England Journal of Medicine*, 318 (March 31, 1988), pp. 797–803.

12. For a defense of the use of age as a standard, see Daniel Callahan, *Setting Limits: Medical Goals in an Aging Society* (New York: Simon and Schuster, 1987); for further discussion of the use of age as a standard, see Paul Homer and Martha Holstein, eds., *Exploring the Limits* (New York: Simon and Schuster, 1990); Timothy M. Smeeding, ed., *Should Medical Care Be Rationed by Age?* (Totowa, N.J.: Rowman and Littlefield, 1987). For some discussions of various efficacy and outcome assess-

ments, see George E. Thibault et al., "Medical Intensive Care: Indications, Interventions, and Outcomes," *Journal of the American Medical Association*, 302 (April 24, 1980), pp. 938–942; Laurence C. Rubenstein et al., "Geriatric Assessment," in *Clinics in Geriatric Medicine*, Vol. 1 (Philadelphia: W. B. Saunders Co., 1987); Andreas Laupacis et al., "An Assessment of Clinically Useful Measures of the Consequences of Treatment," *New England Journal of Medicine*, 318 (June 30, 1988), pp. 1728–1733; Sidney Katz, "Assessing Self Maintenance: Activities of Daily Living, Mobility, and Instrumental Activities of Daily Living," *Journal of the American Geriatrics Society* (December 1983), pp. 721–727; Sidney Katz et al., "Active Life Expectancy," *New England Journal of Medicine*, 309 (November 17, 1983), pp. 1218–1224; Alvan R. Feinstein et al., "Scientific and Clinical Problems in Indexes of Functional Disability," *Annals of Internal Medicine*, 105 (1986), pp. 413–420. See also William B. Schwartz, "The Inevitable Failure of Current Cost-Containment Strategies," *Journal of the American Medical Association*, 257 (January 9, 1987), especially his observation that "the systematic use of so-called benefit curves will be essential to the appropriate allocation of limited resources" (p. 224).

13.     For an acute discussion of the problem of setting limits by individual physician discretion as a way of controlling costs, see Gregory de Lissovoy, "Medicare and Heart Transplants: Will Lightning Strike Twice?" *Health Affairs*, 7 (Fall 1988), pp. 61–72.

14.     Bruce Jennings, "A Grassroots Movement in Bioethics," *Hastings Center Report*, Special Supplement (June/July 1988), pp. 1–16; Louis Harris and Associates, op. cit., pp. 114ff.

15.     There is a large literature on the problems of the physician and rationing or cost containment. See especially Stephen J. McPhee et al., "Cost Containment Confronts Physicians," *Annals of Internal Medicine*, 100 (April 1984), pp. 604–605; David Owen, "Medicine, Morality and the Market," *Canadian Medical Association Journal*, 130 (May 15, 1984), pp. 1341–1345; Marcia Angell, "Cost Containment and the Physician," *Journal of the American Medical Association*, 254 (September 6, 1985), pp. 1203–1207; Gilbert S. Omenn and Douglas A. Conrad, "Implications of DRGs for Physicians," *New England Journal of Medicine*, 311 (November 15, 1984), pp. 1314–1317; Norman Daniels, "Why Saying No to Patients in the United States Is So Hard," *New England Journal of Medicine*, 314 (May 22, 1986), pp. 1380–1383; David Mechanic, "Rationing of Medical Care and the Preservation of Clinical Judgment," *The Journal of Family Practice*, 3 (1980), pp. 431–433; Edmund D. Pellegrino, "Rationing Health Care: The Ethics of Medical Gate Keeping," *Journal of Contemporary Health Law and Policy*, 2 (Spring 1986), pp. 23–45; Michael D. Reagan, "Physicians as Gate Keepers," *New England Journal of Medicine*, 317 (December 31, 1987). For an interesting discussion of the physician's role in the British system, see Rudolf Klein, op. cit., pp. 82ff.

16.     A correction of the malpractice situation in general is imperative for any reform of the American healthcare system: See "Editorial," *Journal of the American Medical Association*, 257 (February 13, 1987), pp. 827–828.

17. The movement to reduce the discrepancy between fees for those in different specialities could be particularly helpful here; cf. William C. Hsiao, "Estimating Physicians' Work for a Resource-Based Relative-Value Scale," *New England Journal of Medicine,* 319 (September 29, 1988), pp. 835–841.

18. The Henry J. Kaiser Family Foundation has organized an imaginative and broad program in health promotion, and the federal government, through its Office of Disease Prevention and Health Promotion, U.S. Public Health Service, has for some years provided important leadership in this area: See *Disease Prevention/Health Promotion: The Facts* (Palo Alto: Bull Publishing Co., 1988); see also Jonathan D. Moreno and Ronald Bayer, "The Limits of the Ledger in Public Health Promotion," *Hastings Center Report* (December 1985), pp. 37–41. For a concrete study of the benefits of a health-promotion strategy, see Theodore Joyce et al., "A Cost-Effectiveness Analysis of Strategies to Reduce Infant Mortality," *Medical Care,* 26 (April 1988), pp. 348–360. For a useful caution on the economic possibilities of saving money through prevention, see Louise B. Russell, *Is Prevention Better than Cure?* (Washington, D.C.: The Brookings Institution, 1986).

19. See especially Ronald Bayer, ed., "Voluntary Health Risks and Public Policy," *Hastings Center Report* (October 1981), pp. 26–44; Daniel I. Wikler, "Persuasion and Coercion for Health," *Milbank Memorial Fund Quarterly,* 56 (1978), pp. 303–338.

20. For a good examination of these issues, see Robert M. Veatch, "Voluntary Risks to Health," *Journal of the American Medical Association,* 243 (January 4, 1980), pp. 50–55; Daniel I. Wikler, "Who Should Be Blamed for Being Sick?" *Health Education Quarterly,* 14 (Spring 1987), pp. 11–25; Robert H. Blank, *Rationing Medicine* (New York: Columbia University Press, 1988), esp. pp. 189ff.

21. For a provocative study of health legislation as an expression of legislative self-interest (that of reelection), see Paul J. Feldstein, *The Politics of Health Legislation* (Ann Arbor: Health Administration Press, 1988).

22. Among the leading proposals for some form of universal health coverage are Uwe E. Reinhardt, "Health Insurance for the Nation's Poor," *Health Affairs,* 6 (Spring 1987); Alain Enthoven and Richard Kronick, "A Consumer-Choice Health Plan for the 1990s," *New England Journal of Medicine,* 2 parts, 320 (January 5, 1989, and January 12, 1989), pp. 29–37, 94–101; David V. Himmelstein et al., "A National Health Program for the United States: A Physician's Proposal," *New England Journal of Medicine,* 320 (January 12, 1989), pp. 102–108; The National Leadership Commission on Health Care, *For the Health of a Nation: A Shared Responsibility* (Washington, D.C.: National Leadership Commission on Health Affairs, January 1989). See also Arnold S. Relman, "Universal Health Insurance: Its Time Has Come," 320 (January 12, 1989), pp. 117–118. The most significant federal legislative initiative to date was the bill introduced by Senators Edward M. Kennedy and Lowell Weicker in the U.S. Senate (S. 1265) in 1987, "Minimum Health Benefits of All Workers Act of 1987"; see also "Massachusetts Health Security Act," which became law in that state on April 21, 1988; R. R. Borbjeng

and C. F. Koller, "State Health Insurance Pools: Current Performance, Future Prospects," *Inquiry*, 23 (1986), pp. 111–121.

23. Alain Enthoven and Richard Kronick, op. cit., p. 31.

24. Ibid.

25. Himmelstein et al., op. cit., p. 102.

26. What, for instance, will be done about the problem of the costs of catastrophic care, about which people can easily be made helplessly cost conscious? The problem of such care poses a dilemma not only for those who will have to bear personally some significant portion of the costs. It will be a critical factor in care for the poor, who will be able to pay little (if any) such costs. For a sobering discussion of this problem, see Marc. L. Berk, Alan C. Monheit, and Michael M. Hagan, "How the U.S. Spent Its Health Care Dollar: 1929–1980," *Health Affairs* (Fall 1988), esp. p. 58. The estimated costs, financial and social, of coping with the AIDS crisis are enormous: See Anne A. Scitovsky, "The Economic Impact of AIDS in the United States," *Health Affairs* (Fall 1988), pp. 32–45; Daniel M. Fox and Emily H. Thomas, "AIDS Cost Analysis and Social Policy," *Law, Medicine and Health Care*, 15 (Winter 1987/88), pp. 186–211.

CHAPTER *8*

1. The poignancy and problems of working at the ragged edge are nicely caught by Thomas Halper, "Life and Death in a Welfare State: End-stage Renal Disease in the United Kingdom," *Milbank Memorial Fund Quarterly*, 63 (1985), pp. 52–93; Albert R. Jonsen, "Bentham in a Box: Technology Assessment and Health Care Technology," *Law, Medicine and Health Care*, 14 (1986), pp. 172–174.

2. Three recent books that fully develop the case for active euthanasia and assisted suicide are James Rachels, *The End of Life: Euthanasia and Morality* (New York: Oxford University Press, 1986); Helga Kuhse, *The Sanctity-of-Life Doctrine in Medicine: A Critique* (Oxford: Oxford University Press, 1987), esp. Chap. 2; Derek Humphrey and Ann Wickett, *The Right to Die: Understanding Euthanasia* (New York: Harper and Row, 1986). See also John Arras, "The Right to Die on a Slippery Slope," *Social Theory and Practice*, 8 (Fall 1982), pp. 285–328.

3. See Mark Siegler, "Should Age Be a Criterion in Health Care?" *Hastings Center Report*, 14 (October 1984), p. 26.

4. For an interesting analysis of the possible reasons for the failure of the California referendum initiative, see Alan Parachini, "The California Humane and Dignified Death Initiative," in *Mercy, Murder and Morality: Perspectives on Euthanasia*, a special supplement of the *Hastings Center Report* (January/February 1989), pp. 10–11.

5. For analyses of the Dutch situation, see Richard Fenigsen, "A Case Against Dutch Euthanasia," and Hengt Rigter, "Euthanasia in the

Netherlands: Distinguishing Facts from Fiction," both in *Mercy, Murder and Morality: Perspectives on Euthanasia.*

6.   Louis Harris, *Inside America* (New York: Vintage Books, 1987), pp. 154–155; see also Susan Waller, "Trends in Public Acceptance of Euthanasia Worldwide," *The Euthanasia Review* (Spring 1986), pp. 333–347.

7.   J. Lubitz and R. Prihoda, "Uses and Costs of Medicare Services in the Last Two Years of Life," *Health Care Financing Review*, 5 (Spring 1984), pp. 117–131.

8.   Anne A. Scitovsky, " 'The High Cost of Dying': What Do the Data Show," *Milbank Memorial Fund Quarterly*, 62 (1984), pp. 591–608; Anne A. Scitovsky, "Medical Care in the Last Twelve Months of Life: The Relationship between Age, Functional Status and Medical Care Expenditures," unpublished paper, May 1988; Noralov P. Roos et al., "Health Care Utilization in the Years Prior to Death," *The Milbank Quarterly*, 65 (1987), pp. 231–254.

9.   A. S. Detsky et al., "Prognosis, Survival, and the Expenditure of Hospital Patients in an Intensive-Care Unit," *New England Journal of Medicine*, 305 (1981), p. 668.

10.  Jessica H. Muller and Barbara A. Koenig, "On the Boundary of Life and Death: The Definition of Dying by Medical Residents," in Margaret Lock and Deborah Gordon, eds., *Biomedicine Examined* (Dordrecht: Kluwer Academic Publishers, 1988), p. 369.

11.  For a full treatment of this view, see Charles J. McFadden, *Medical Ethics* (Philadelphia: F. A. Davis, 1968), Chaps. 10 and 11.

12.  Yale Kamisar, "Some Non-Religious Views Against Proposed Mercy-Killing Legislation," *Human Life Review*, Parts I and II (Spring and Summer 1976), pp. 71–114 (I) and pp. 34–63 (II); see also Germain Grisez and Joseph M. Boyle, Jr., *Life and Death with Liberty and Justice* (Notre Dame, Ind.: University of Notre Dame Press, 1979).

13.  Robert Jay Lifton, *The Nazi Doctors: Medical Killing and the Psychology of Genocide* (New York: Basic Books, 1986), esp. Part I; see also Gary E. Crum, "Nazi Bioethics and a Doctor's Defense," *Human Life Review*, 8 (Summer 1982), pp. 55–69; "Biomedical Ethics and the Shadow of Nazism," a special supplement of the *Hastings Center Report* (August 1976).

14.  Earlier versions of this argument appeared in Daniel Callahan, "Can We Return Death to Disease?" *Hastings Center Report*, 19 (January/February 1989), special supplement, pp. 4–6, and in "Vital Distinctions, Mortal Questions," *Commonweal* (July 15, 1988), pp. 397–404.

15.  John Stuart Mill, "On Liberty," in Mary Warnock, ed., *John Stuart Mill, Utilitarianism* (Cleveland and New York: Meridan, 1962), p. 236.

16.  The traditional distinction is challenged at length by both James Rachels, op. cit., and Helga Kuhse, op. cit.; for a criticism of Rachels's view that goes in a somewhat different direction than mine, see Tom L. Beauchamp, "A Reply to Rachels on Active and Passive Euthanasia,"

in Tom L. Beauchamp and Seymour Perlin, eds., *Ethical Issues in Death and Dying* (Englewood Cliffs, N.J.: Prentice-Hall, 1978), pp. 246–258.

17. Dan W. Brock, "Forgoing Life-Sustaining Food and Water: Is It Killing?" in Joanne Lynn, ed., *By No Extraordinary Means: The Choice to Forgo Food and Water* (Bloomington, Ind.: Indiana University Press, 1986), p. 126. Brock's article is a particularly valuable discussion of these issues.

18. A good discussion of the distinction between withholding and withdrawing treatment can be found in the Hastings Center, *Guidelines on the Termination of Life-Sustaining Treatment and the Care of the Dying* (Briarcliff Manor, N.Y.: The Hastings Center, 1987), pp. 130–131; see also President's Commission for the Study of Ethical Problems in Medicine and Biomedical and Behavioral Research, *Deciding to Forgo Life-Sustaining Treatment* (Washington, D.C.: Government Printing Office, 1983), p. 73.

19. Albert Jonsen effectively reviews a variety of traditional and other objections to physicians carrying out active euthanasia in "Beyond the Physician's Reference—The Ethics of Active Euthanasia," *Western Journal of Medicine,* 149 (August 1988), pp. 195–198; also Willard Gaylin et al., "Doctors Must Not Kill, *Journal of the American Medical Association,* 2259 (April 8, 1988), pp. 2139–2140.

20. This view seems strongly reflected in William E. May et al., "Feeding and Hydrating the Permanently Unconscious and Other Vulnerable Persons," *Issues in Law and Medicine,* 3 (Winter 1987), pp. 203–217.

21. This possibility was foreshadowed by Roger Evans, "Health Care Technology and the Inevitability of Resource Allocation and Rationing Decisions," Part 2, *Journal of the American Medical Association,* 249 (April 22/29, 1983), p. 2217.

22. Nat Hentoff, "The 'Small Beginnings' of Death," *The Human Life Review,* 14 (Spring 1988), pp. 53–88.

23. For example, the *Guidelines on the Termination of Life-Sustaining Treatment and the Care of the Dying,* op. cit., and Stephen F. Miles and Carlos F. Gomez, *Protocols for Elective Use of Life-Sustaining Treatments* (New York: Springer, 1989); see also Cynthia Cohen, ed., *Casebook on the Termination of Life-Sustaining Treatment and the Care of the Dying* (Bloomington: Indiana University Press, 1988).

24. See Nancy K. Rhoden, "Litigating Life and Death," *Harvard Law Review,* 102 (December 1988), pp. 375–446.

CHAPTER 9

1. Antoine-Nicolas de Condorcet, *Sketch for a Historical Picture of the Progress of the Human Mind,* trans. by June Berraclough (New York: Library of Ideas, 1955), p. 200. I was reminded of this passage while reading Gerald J. Gruman's remarkable monograph "A History of Ideas about the Prolongation of Life," *Transactions of the American Philosophical Society,* 56 (Part 9, 1966).

2. Lewis Thomas, "On the Science and Technology of Medicine," *Daedalus* (Winter 1977), p. 46. Hiroshi Nakajima, "Address to the All-Union Conference of Physicians," WHO Press, Press Release WHO/37 (October 18, 1988).

3. Michael Ignatieff, "Modern Dying," *New Republic* (December 26, 1988), p. 32.

4. René Dubos, *Mirage of Health: Utopias, Progress, and Biological Change* (New York: Harper Colophon Books, 1979), p. 2.

5. Michael Walzer, *Spheres of Justice: A Defense of Pluralism and Equality* (New York: Basic Books, 1983), p. 8.

6. Ignatieff, op. cit., p. 31.

7. Robert G. Evans, "Finding the Levers, Finding the Courage: Lessons from Cost Containment in North America," *Journal of Health Politics, Policy and Law*, 11 (1986), p. 600.

8. While it may represent an unusually pessimistic view of the Canadian system, see Michael A. Walker, "Neighborly Advice on Health Care," *Wall Street Journal* (June 8, 1988), p. 18. A more optimistic view can be found in Robert G. Evans, " 'We'll Take Care of It for You'—Health Care in the Canadian Community," *Daedalus*, 117 (Fall 1988), pp. 155–189.

9. Rudolf Klein, *The Politics of the National Health Service* (New York: Longman, 1983), p. 182.

# INDEX